# WHO Health Evidence Network synthesis report 68

# What is the current alcohol labelling practice in the WHO European Region and what are barriers and facilitators to development and implementation of alcohol labelling policy?

Eva Jané-Llopis | Daša Kokole | Maria Neufeld |
Omer Syed Muhammad Hasan | Jürgen Rehm

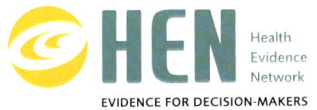

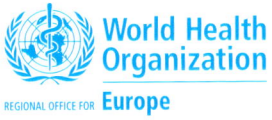

## Abstract

The WHO European Region has the highest levels of alcohol consumption per capita in the world, yet alcohol labelling, a WHO-recommended practice that provides consumer information on the ingredients, nutritional values and harms of alcohol, is not mandatory. This report synthesizes evidence on alcohol labelling practices in the Region and aims to describe factors affecting implementation. To date, the introduction of alcohol labelling policy as part of a larger package of alcohol policy measures created with strong political support and consumer pressure has proved successful in providing consumers with information, although practices have been hindered by slow procedures in some parts of the Region, opposition from international institutions and the alcohol industry, and the lack of set labelling specifications and monitoring activities. Policy considerations for the development of successful labelling legislation should ideally address both health information and nutritional information, ensure regulated message presentation and implement independent monitoring and evaluation of measures.

### Keywords
ALCOHOL CONSUMPTION, CONSUMER HEALTH INFORMATION, FOOD LABELLING, NUTRITIONAL VALUE, HEALTH PROMOTION

---

Address requests about publications of the WHO Regional Office for Europe to:
 Publications
 WHO Regional Office for Europe
 UN City, Marmorvej 51
 DK-2100 Copenhagen Ø, Denmark
Alternatively, complete an online request form for documentation, health information, or for permission to quote or translate, on the Regional Office website (http://www.euro.who.int/pubrequest).

---

ISSN 2227-4316
ISBN 978 92 890 5489 8

### © World Health Organization 2020

Some rights reserved. This work is available under the Creative Commons Attribution-NonCommercial-ShareAlike 3.0 IGO licence (CC BY-NC-SA 3.0 IGO; https://creativecommons.org/licenses/by-nc-sa/3.0/igo).

Under the terms of this licence, you may copy, redistribute and adapt the work for non-commercial purposes, provided the work is appropriately cited, as indicated below. In any use of this work, there should be no suggestion that WHO endorses any specific organization, products or services. The use of the WHO logo is not permitted. If you adapt the work, then you must license your work under the same or equivalent Creative Commons licence. If you create a translation of this work, you should add the following disclaimer along with the suggested citation: "This translation was not created by the World Health Organization (WHO). WHO is not responsible for the content or accuracy of this translation. The original English edition shall be the binding and authentic edition".

Any mediation relating to disputes arising under the licence shall be conducted in accordance with the mediation rules of the World Intellectual Property Organization.

**Suggested citation.** Jané-Llopis E, Kokole D, Neufeld M, Hasan OSM, Rehm J. What is the current alcohol labelling practice in the WHO European Region and what are barriers and facilitators to development and implementation of alcohol labelling policy? Copenhagen: WHO Regional Office for Europe; 2020 (Health Evidence Network (HEN) synthesis report 68).

**Cataloguing-in-Publication (CIP) data.** CIP data are available at http://apps.who.int/iris.

**Sales, rights and licensing.** To purchase WHO publications, see http://apps.who.int/bookorders. To submit requests for commercial use and queries on rights and licensing, see http://www.who.int/about/licensing.

**Third-party materials.** If you wish to reuse material from this work that is attributed to a third party, such as tables, figures or images, it is your responsibility to determine whether permission is needed for that reuse and to obtain permission from the copyright holder. The risk of claims resulting from infringement of any third-party-owned component in the work rests solely with the user.

**General disclaimers.** The designations employed and the presentation of the material in this publication do not imply the expression of any opinion whatsoever on the part of WHO concerning the legal status of any country, territory, city or area or of its authorities, or concerning the delimitation of its frontiers or boundaries. Dotted and dashed lines on maps represent approximate border lines for which there may not yet be full agreement.

The mention of specific companies or of certain manufacturers' products does not imply that they are endorsed or recommended by WHO in preference to others of a similar nature that are not mentioned. Errors and omissions excepted, the names of proprietary products are distinguished by initial capital letters.

All reasonable precautions have been taken by WHO to verify the information contained in this publication. However, the published material is being distributed without warranty of any kind, either expressed or implied. The responsibility for the interpretation and use of the material lies with the reader. In no event shall WHO be liable for damages arising from its use.

The named authors alone are responsible for the views expressed in this publication.

Printed in Luxembourg

# CONTENTS

▸ Abbreviations ................................................................................................. iv

▸ Acknowledgements ......................................................................................... v

▸ Summary ...................................................................................................... viii

▸ 1. Introduction ................................................................................................ 1
   ▸ 1.1 Background .......................................................................................... 1
   ▸ 1.2 Methodology ........................................................................................ 5

▸ 2. Results ......................................................................................................... 7
   ▸ 2.1 National legislation on labelling for alcoholic beverages ................... 7
   ▸ 2.2 Industry-led voluntary commitments on labelling
       for alcoholic beverages ........................................................................ 13
   ▸ 2.3 Monitoring implementation of alcohol labelling ............................... 15
   ▸ 2.4 Alignment of labelling practices with WHO recommendations ........ 22
   ▸ 2.5 Factors supporting the development and implementation
       of regulatory frameworks for alcohol labelling .................................. 23
   ▸ 2.6 Factors hindering the development and implementation
       of regulatory frameworks for alcohol labelling .................................. 28

▸ 3. Discussion .................................................................................................. 36
   ▸ 3.1 Strengths and limitations of this review ............................................. 36
   ▸ 3.2 Ensuring the rights to consumer information through labelling ..... 37
   ▸ 3.3 Ensuring adequate and independent monitoring ............................. 38
   ▸ 3.4 Policy considerations ......................................................................... 39

▸ 4. Conclusions ............................................................................................... 41

▸ References .................................................................................................... 42

▸ Annex 1. Search strategy ............................................................................. 63

▸ Annex 2. Nutritional and health information labelling legislation
   and commitments for countries and industries ........................................ 68

# ABBREVIATIONS

CMO     Chief Medical Officer (United Kingdom)
EU      European Union

# ACKNOWLEDGEMENTS

The authors would like to thank all the Member State representatives who participated in the regional consultation organized in January 2019 by the WHO Regional Office for Europe and to acknowledge their valuable contributions to this report. We thank Professor Peter Anderson for his input through the different phases of the manuscript. We also thank Catherine Bernard, Eunan McKinney, Mariann Skar, Stig Erik Sørheim, Ismo Tuominen and Wim van Dalen and the Alcohol Prevention Team in the Scottish Government and Public Health England for reviewing parts of text and providing further country-specific information.

This report and all the activities related to it were made possible due to the financial support provided by the Government of Germany, the Government of Norway and the Government of the Russian Federation in the context of the WHO European Office for the Prevention and Control of Noncommunicable Diseases.

## Authors

Eva Jané-Llopis
Director, Health, SDGs and Social Innovation, Ramon Llull University, ESADE Business School, Barcelona, Spain; Senior Associate Professor, Care and Public Health Research Institute, Maastricht University, Maastricht, the Netherlands; and Senior Scientist, Institute for Mental Health Policy Research, Centre for Addiction and Mental Health, Toronto, Canada

Daša Kokole
Researcher, Department of Health Promotion, CAPHRI Care and Public Health Research Institute, Maastricht University, Maastricht, the Netherlands

Maria Neufeld
Doctoral candidate, Institute for Clinical Psychology and Psychotherapy, Technische Universität Dresden, Dresden, Germany

Omer Syed Muhammad Hasan
Research Methods Specialist, Institute for Mental Health Policy Research, Centre for Addiction and Mental Health, Toronto, Canada

Jürgen Rehm
Professor, Department of International Health Projects, Institute for Leadership and Health Management, I.M. Sechenov First Moscow State Medical University, Moscow, the Russian Federation; Senior Scientist, Institute for Mental Health Policy Research, Centre for Addiction and Mental Health, Toronto, Canada; and Professor, Dalla Lana School of Public Health and Department of Psychiatry, University of Toronto, Toronto, Canada

Peer reviewers

Erin Hobin
Scientist, Public Health Ontario and Dalla Lana School of Public Health, University of Toronto, Toronto, and Centre for Substance Use Research, University of Victoria, Victoria, Canada

Aleksandra Kaczmarek
Policy Manager, European Alcohol Policy Alliance, Brussels, Belgium

Jose M Martin-Moreno
Professor of Preventive Medicine and Public Health, University of Valencia, and INCLIVA Instituto de Investigación Sanitaria, Valencia, Spain

Editorial team, WHO Regional Office for Europe

Division of Noncommunicable Diseases and Promoting Health through the Life-course

Joao Breda
Head, WHO European Office for the Prevention and Control of Noncommunicable Diseases

Carina Ferreira-Borges
Programme Manager, Alcohol and Illicit Drugs, WHO European Office for the Prevention and Control of Noncommunicable Diseases

Bente Mikkelsen
Director, Noncommunicable Diseases and Promoting Health through the Life-course, WHO Regional Office for Europe

Health Evidence Network (HEN) editorial team

Kristina Mauer-Stender, Acting Director
Tanja Kuchenmüller, Editor in Chief
Tarang Sharma and Ryoko Takahashi, Series Editors
Tyrone Reden Sy, Managing Editor
Krista Kruja, Consultant
Jane Ward, Technical Editor

The HEN Secretariat is part of the Division of Information, Evidence, Research and Innovation at the WHO Regional Office for Europe. HEN synthesis reports are commissioned works that are subjected to international peer review, and the contents are the responsibility of the authors. They do not necessarily reflect the official policies of the Regional Office.

# SUMMARY

## The issue

The WHO European Region has the highest levels of per capita alcohol consumption worldwide, with 10% of all deaths attributable to alcohol. Alcohol labelling, a WHO-recommended practice, is in line with principles of consumer protection and safety through providing consumers with information about alcohol risks. To date, there is no overview on the presence of mandatory or voluntary nutritional value, ingredients listing and health information labelling on alcoholic beverages in the Region, nor the factors influencing labelling practice.

## The synthesis question

This report reviews the evidence on existing practices for nutritional and health information labelling on alcoholic products to address the question: "What is the current alcohol labelling practice in the WHO European Region and what are barriers and facilitators to development and implementation of alcohol labelling policy?"

## Types of evidence

A scoping review was undertaken to identify academic and grey literature from the WHO European Region in 14 languages (Bosnian, Catalan, Croatian, Dutch, English, French, German, Italian, Montenegrin, Romanian, Russian, Serbian, Slovene and Spanish). From the 6988 documents screened, a final total of 124 documents were included in the report.

## Results

In the WHO European Region, 40% of Member States have some legislation on ingredients listing, 19% have some legislation on inclusion of nutritional values and 28% have some legislation on some health information labelling or warnings on alcohol products (including warnings for pregnant women, on drinking and driving and on underage drinking or general warnings on harm to health). Compared with other fields, such as tobacco or foodstuffs, the presence of labelling on alcohol products is limited and most labelling legislation still does not align fully with WHO's 2017 discussion paper on policy options for alcohol labelling (*Alcohol labelling: a discussion document on policy options*), particularly with regards to presentation of the label (in terms of message size and visibility and periodically changing the nature of the message (rotating messages)).

Voluntary industry commitments vary in scope, in the information included across product categories and in how the information is displayed. Commitments are mostly not monitored transparently and, where available, do not meet recommendations in the WHO discussion paper on policy options for alcohol labelling.

The main factors influencing the successful implementation of legislation regarding alcohol labelling have been its introduction as part of a larger package of strict alcohol-related policy measures, strong political support and consumer pressure. Labelling practice has often been hindered by slow procedures in some parts of the Region, opposition from international bodies and their members, opposition and lobbying from the alcohol industry, lack of precise specifications for the label, and lack of monitoring and enforcement activities.

The existence of legislation or a commitment does not ensure implementation is enforced nor that it has the expected reach. Except for one European Union (EU)-wide study, little independent monitoring of the presence of messages on labels of alcoholic beverages or the impact of different message types could be identified regardless of whether the labelling was mandatory or voluntary.

## Policy considerations

Based on the findings of this review, the main policy and practice considerations in the WHO European Region for the development of nutritional and health information labelling on alcohol products are to:

- establish labelling that includes all recommended nutritional values and lists all ingredients;
- establish labelling that includes the harm done by alcohol relevant to the whole population (e.g. cancer), pregnancy-related harm, harm to minors, drinking and driving warnings, and recommendations on lower-risk drinking guidelines indicated as standard drinks in countries where this would be applicable;
- ensure regulations include specific directions about how all information should be presented on labels (e.g. appropriate size and font, front of pack, rotating messages and easy-to-understand information), ideally following WHO recommendations;
- favour mandatory regulation over voluntary commitments as this allows better control over the content and presentation of the message, presentation of stronger evidence and more assurance of good penetration of labelling;

- provide clear input and direction from public health bodies if messages are to be voluntary and self-regulated by industry to ensure that effective messages are displayed;
- consider introducing any specific labelling policy as a part of an existing or new, larger policy package and using a stepwise approach to facilitate achieving a full labelling policy;
- leverage facilitating contextual factors when developing policy (e.g. public support, political will and/or evidence of alcohol-related harm in the country) and use the best policy window to put proposals forward for the introduction of labelling;
- expect some barriers to the development of legislation, such as opposition from the alcohol industry or delays in processes of international bodies, and have strong counterarguments prepared in advance to best support the proposed legislation;
- ensure that mechanisms for enforcing implementation, for independent monitoring and for evaluation of the impact of labelling policies are in place regardless of whether labelling is voluntary or mandatory; and
- invest in strengthening research on alcohol labelling to identify the most effective form and content of the labelling communication (e.g. photographs, pictograms and written messages, including the most effective wording).

# 1. INTRODUCTION

## 1.1 Background

### 1.1.1 Alcohol as a public health problem

Alcohol is an intoxicating substance with negative consequences for the individual and society. Use of alcohol ranks as the seventh leading global risk factor for ill health and premature death (1). In 2016 alcohol use was the cause of over 900 000 deaths in the WHO European Region (2,3) and about 3 million deaths worldwide (1,2). The WHO European Region continues to have the highest levels of per capita alcohol consumption (9.8 litres of pure alcohol per year) and, globally, the highest proportion of burden of disease attributable to alcohol, with 10.1% of all deaths and 10.8% of all disability-adjusted life-years attributable to alcohol consumption (2).

Alcohol causes cancers of the oral cavity and pharynx, oesophagus, stomach, colon, rectum and breast (in females) (4,5). Chronic and irregular heavy drinking is detrimental to cardiovascular health, being related to hypertension, ischaemic heart disease and stroke (6). Even moderate alcohol use increases blood pressure and stroke risk (7). Alcohol consumption also increases the risk of communicable diseases (e.g. tuberculosis, HIV/AIDS), partly through its effects on decision-making and behaviours and partly through its immunosuppressant properties (8,9). It is also linked with a range of mental health disorders, including depression (10,11). The threshold for lowest risk should be lower than that commonly applied in low-risk drinking guidelines, at about 100 grams (125 ml) of alcohol per week (i.e. 12.5 units) (12), noting that no level of alcohol consumption is safe (13). For most diseases, there is a dose–response relationship, with the risk becoming higher with the more alcohol consumed, and often increasing exponentially (6).

Alcohol also impacts on the social environment, for example through increased criminal and aggressive behaviour and violence (14,15). The estimated societal costs of alcohol in the EU in 2003 was calculated at €125 billion in tangible costs (health care, treatment, crime, traffic accidents and productivity losses), and a further €270 billion in intangible costs (e.g. pain, suffering and years of healthy life lost) (16). The costs of alcohol use have been estimated to be higher than those of all illicit drugs combined and similar to the costs of tobacco (17).

### 1.1.2 Evidence for labelling effectiveness

Similar to smoking and obesity, alcohol consumption is a complex system-level issue influenced by various interconnected individual, societal and environmental factors (18). Therefore, shifting population-level alcohol use will require a comprehensive strategy, including increasing taxation, a reduction of availability, a ban on advertising and marketing, and the introduction of product labelling. These measures are part of both the WHO *European action plan to reduce the harmful use of alcohol 2012–2020* (19) and the WHO *Global strategy to reduce the harmful use of alcohol* (20), which call for "provision of consumer information about, and labelling of, alcoholic beverages to indicate the harm related to alcohol". Such consumer information can, in turn, increase public support for more stringent policies, such as taxation and are, therefore, an important part of an overall alcohol policy package (21).

The strongest evidence of labelling effectiveness is in the areas of nutrition and tobacco, where labelling is mandatory. Nutritional labelling has been found to lead to changes in consumer behaviour, both by increasing the number of people selecting a healthier product (22) and by reducing consumer dietary intake of unhealthy options (23). Nutritional labelling also has been found to influence industry responses, leading to changes in the composition of some products (23). Health information labelling in tobacco products has shown that labels can be effective in promoting smoking cessation and preventing smoking uptake by young people; that graphic/pictogram warning labels, taking up a large portion of front of packages, with rotating messages to prevent adaptation are most effective (24); and that overall warnings increase knowledge and reduce smoking behaviour (25).

There has been less research on the effectiveness of labels for alcohol. Some older reviews found that warning labels in the United States of America had limited impact on drinking behaviour but did lead to an increase in awareness of the messages (26–28). Pictorial warnings can raise awareness and understanding of the risks of alcohol consumption: general ("alcohol increases your risk of cancer") compared with specific ("alcohol increases your risk of breast cancer") messages are perceived as more believable and convincing, as are qualitative messages compared with quantitative ones (29). A 2017 meta-analysis found medium effect sizes for consumers in remembering warning labels, but enhanced impact when the message is made explicit, rather than inferred or requiring the consumer to translate numbers into a given risk (30). Labels with standard drink information and low-risk drinking guidelines are effective for helping drinkers to accurately estimate their alcohol consumption (31–33) and have the support of the public (33,34). Consequently, although this is an understudied area, the available evidence for alcohol labelling remains relatively favourable (35) and supports the use of practices closer to those for tobacco in particular (24) and, to a large extent, food products (36), where evidence is irrefutable.

The introduction of alcohol labelling has been shown to be more effective if it is part of a broader package of alcohol policies, including depiction of the consequences of alcohol consumption, and broader social communication campaigns that aim to foster long-term changes in society's perception, attitudes and social norms around alcohol (18,37,38). The effectiveness of this packaged approach has been demonstrated for both tobacco and nutrition, where warning labels are often not a standalone practice but are accompanied by other policy measures (26,39).

Mandatory labelling already exists for similar consumer products, such as non-alcoholic beverages. Alcoholic beverages fall under the definition of food (40) in the labelling-related provisions of the Codex Alimentarius Commission[1] standards and guidelines (41,42), and so are not exempted from the obligatory listing of all their ingredients and nutrient declaration (43). Yet, this has not been clearly understood by its Member States (40) and discussions around standards and procedures for labelling alcohol products within the Commission are still ongoing. Countries are not in agreement as to whether to devote special attention to alcohol labelling separately from food labelling and, if so, which alcohol labelling issues (e.g. alcohol content, nutritional information) should be considered (40). This is not surprising in that there are 186 Member States of the Commission, with variations in experienced level of harm caused by alcohol and in existing alcohol labelling practices. Consequently, lengthy discussions will be needed to devise a solution that would be relevant for all Member States.

### 1.1.3 What should be displayed on labels?

There is also debate regarding what information on alcohol should be displayed and how information should be conveyed to consumers, for example through ingredients listing, nutritional information and/or health information. A review in 2013 of enhanced labelling on alcoholic drinks to guide alcohol policy identified five elements as useful to consumers: list of ingredients, nutritional information, serving size and servings per container, a definition of moderate intake and health information (44).

---

[1] The Codex Alimentarius Commission is the Joint WHO/Food and Agriculture Organization of the United Nations body that produces internationally adopted food standards and guidelines intended to facilitate international trade and promote food safety and public health.

Further, the proven detrimental effects of alcohol on health (e.g. high caloric value (45), potential obesogenic role (46–55) and related burden (56), and carcinogenic and mutagenic effects (57,58)) and the general lack of public awareness of these has resulted in calls for stringent labelling that includes all nutritional information and health-related information (59), with content suggestions (60,61) mirroring tobacco warning labels. The WHO 2017 discussion paper on policy options for alcohol labelling (62) suggested that alcohol labelling should include specific features (Box 1).

Box 1. WHO options for product labelling
- Include a list of ingredients, including nutritional values on containers: energy, amounts of total fat, saturated fat, carbohydrates, sugars, protein and salt.
- Provide information on labels explaining impact on health (e.g. cancer).
- Provide labels with the following characteristics:
  - placed in a standard location on the container;
  - size determined as a minimum percentage of the size of the container;
  - with rotating messages (to prevent adaptation to the content of the message);
  - with clear separation of text from other information;
  - with text printed in capital letters and bold type, appearing on a contrasting background and written in the official language of the country where the product is sold;
  - with informational images taken from ongoing education campaigns; and
  - based on advice from public health bodies on the content of the messages.

Source: WHO, 2017 (62).

Both the 2017 *Alcohol labelling: discussion document on policy options* (62) and the 2011 *European action plan to reduce the harmful use of alcohol* (19) from the WHO Regional Office for Europe recommend including both nutritional information and health-related information on the labels. Aligning with the requirements of EU regulation No. 1169/2011 for non-alcoholic beverage packaging (63), the policy discussion document recommended that alcohol packaging include a list of ingredients and nutritional values. For alcohol's impact on health, the policy discussion document called for messages including the general health effects of alcohol (e.g. cancer), pregnancy-related harm, harm to minors, drinking and driving warnings and lower-risk drinking guidelines.

The focus for alcohol labelling should be on both the content of the message and its clear presentation. Health Evidence Network synthesis report 61 on front-of-packaging labelling found that consumer use and understanding of labelling was poor, particularly in disadvantaged populations, because of the complexity of the numerical information, small print size and positioning on the back or side of packs (36). The report highlighted the importance of adopting a single front-of-pack labelling system for supporting consumer label use and understanding.

### 1.1.4 Objectives of this report

While reviews on alcohol labelling have been undertaken (26,35,64–67), none to date has systematically reviewed labelling implementation in all the Member States of the WHO European Region. This scoping review encompasses the whole Region, examining legislation, industry-led voluntary measures, and barriers and facilitators for policy development and implementation; it also derives policy considerations to strengthen alcohol labelling.

Based on the recommendations in the 2017 WHO discussion paper on policy options for alcohol labelling (62), the following characteristics of labels were assessed in existing practice:

- for nutritional information labelling:
  - list of ingredients on the label
  - list of nutritional values on the label
- for health information labelling:
  - any health- or harm-related messages on the label
  - specification of the messages (e.g. size and visibility).

The WHO terminology of health information labelling has been used in this report, rather than that of health warnings, although many published articles and many countries use the latter terminology.

## 1.2 Methodology

A literature search between September and November 2018 (with updated searches in May and June 2019) examined peer-reviewed and grey literature on the presence and implementation of existing alcohol labelling policies and voluntary commitments, and their evaluation, specifically when highlighting hindering and facilitating factors. Documents were identified from all 53 Member States of the WHO European

Region and in 14 languages (Bosnian, Catalan, Croatian, Dutch, English, French, German, Italian, Montenegrin, Romanian, Russian, Serbian, Slovene and Spanish).

The search of the peer-reviewed literature identified 1592 articles after removal of duplicates; 20 full-text articles were reviewed, with eight fulfilling the criteria for inclusion (68–75). The search of the grey literature identified 5396 articles, with 299 selected for full-text review and 116 finally included (63,76–190). Data were also used from the WHO Global Information System on Alcohol and Health (191). Further details on the search strategy are provided in Annex 1.

## 2. RESULTS

All the results in this section derive from the WHO European Region unless specified as from elsewhere.

### 2.1 National legislation on labelling for alcoholic beverages

Table 1 gives an overview of national alcohol labelling legislation in the WHO European Region, as discussed below.

Labelling regulations were more likely to mandate the inclusion of listing ingredients (40% of Member States) as opposed to information on nutritional values (19% of Member States; all included ingredients listing). Considering the inclusion of both an ingredients list and nutritional values, only 19% of WHO European Region Member States comply with the recommendations made in the WHO discussion paper on policy options for alcohol labelling (62). Non-EU Member

Table 1. Presence of nutritional and health information in alcohol labelling legislation in the WHO European Region, overall and by EU membership

| Countries/Region | Ingredients | | Nutritional values[a] | | Health information | | All three | |
|---|---|---|---|---|---|---|---|---|
| | n | % | n | % | n | % | n | % |
| WHO European Region (overall) | 21 | 40 | 10 | 19 | 15 | 28 | 9 | 17 |
| EU Member States (28) | 9 | 32 | 1 | 4 | 4 | 14 | 1 | 4 |
| Non-EU Members States (25) | 12 | 48 | 9 | 36 | 11 | 44 | 8 | 32 |

[a] All countries with legislation on including nutritional values also had legislation on including an ingredients list.

States meet the recommendations in more than one third of cases (36%), whereas only one EU Member State (4%) is compliant with the recommendations in full.

In terms of health information labelling, 28% of the WHO European Region Member States have introduced legislation to include some form of health-related information on the label, thus meeting WHO suggestions in the discussion paper on policy options for alcohol labelling. More non-EU Member States have health information legislation (44%) than do EU Member States (14%).

### 2.1.1 Nutritional labelling legislation

Fig. 1 depicts the 21 countries that have nutritional labelling legislation in place mandating ingredients, nutritional value or both (68,76–79). Table A2.1 in Annex 2 provides the specific legislation and the types of nutritional information required in each country.

Fig. 1. Member States with nutritional information legislation on alcohol labels

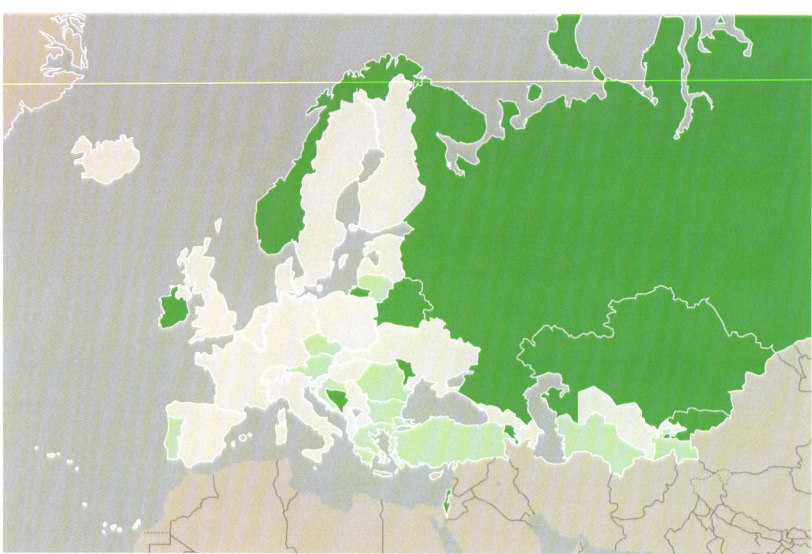

Requirements predominantly pertain to disclosing the list of all ingredients, as currently is the case in 21 countries (Armenia, Austria, Belarus, Bosnia and Herzegovina, Bulgaria, Croatia, Czechia, Greece, Ireland, Israel, Kazakhstan, Kyrgyzstan, Lithuania, Norway, Portugal, Republic of Moldova, Romania, the Russian Federation, Tajikistan, Turkey and Turkmenistan). Some of the countries (Austria, Bulgaria and Republic of Moldova) only have this requirement for beer. Nutritional value declaration is only required in 10 countries (Armenia, Belarus, Bosnia and Herzegovina, Ireland, Israel, Kazakhstan, Kyrgyzstan, Norway, Republic of Moldova (only for beer) and the Russian Federation). Five of these (Armenia, Belarus, Kazakhstan, Kyrgyzstan and the Russian Federation) form the Eurasian Economic Union and are bound by a joint technical regulation (Box 2). Ireland and Norway only passed the legislation in 2018, with implementation still to start. Ireland, with its recently passed Public Health (Alcohol) Bill (152), is the first, and so far the only, EU Member State that has the requirement for listing the energy value (expressed in kilojoules and kilocalories) for alcoholic beverages.

> **Box 2. Technical regulations in the Eurasian Economic Union**
>
> In 2011 the Eurasian Customs Union (Belarus, Kazakhstan and the Russian Federation) adopted the Technical regulation on food products labelling (TR SU 022/2011) (89) and the Technical regulation on food safety (TR SU 021/2011) (90), which prescribed safety requirements for any foodstuff products, including alcoholic beverages, and obliged countries to include a list of ingredients and nutritional value on the label. The legislation was amended in 2013 and 2014 (91) and Member States were given until January 2016 to implement any required changes (92).
>
> In 2011 the Eurasian Customs Union also drafted a Technical regulation on safety of alcoholic beverages in addition to the already implemented regulations on food safety and labelling. This new regulation required an additional health information message "Excessive consumption of alcohol harms your health", which would cover at least 20% of the label, and the following recommendation: "Alcohol use is not recommended for persons under the age of 21, pregnant and lactating women, as well as persons with diseases of the nervous system and internal organs" (93). The draft regulation was notified to neighbouring countries for comments through the World Trade Organization in 2015 (94) and, with some changes, it was finally agreed in December 2018. In its final version, the regulation required the health information message "Excessive consumption of alcohol harms your health" covering at least 10% of the

Box 2 contd

label and the following information on the packaging: "Alcohol use is not recommended for persons under the age of 18, pregnant and lactating women, as well as persons with diseases of the nervous system and internal organs". However, for alcoholic beverages sold on the territory of the Republic of Kazakhstan, the following health information message needed to be placed on the label: "Alcohol is contraindicated for persons under the age of 21, pregnant and lactating women, persons with diseases of the central nervous system, kidneys, liver and digestive organs." In line with the general regulations of the Eurasian Economic Union, this adopted Technical regulation will come into force in January 2021, following a two-year transition period (80).

During the different phases of the regulation process, the Eurasian Customs Union was incorporated in the Eurasian Economic Union's legal framework and expanded its membership, with Armenia and Kyrgyzstan joining Belarus, Kazakhstan and the Russian Federation in 2015. By joining, the new members were subjected to requirements of the nutritional information-related technical regulations accepted in previous years (Technical regulation on food products labelling and Technical regulation on food safety). Likewise, all members will have to implement the recently passed health information-related labelling regulations (Technical regulation on safety of alcoholic beverages), superseding any previous national regulations.

### 2.1.2 Health information legislation

Fig. 2 depicts the 15 countries that have introduced some form of health information legislation (76,80–88): Armenia, Belarus, France, Germany, Ireland, Israel, Kazakhstan, Kyrgyzstan, Lithuania, Norway, Republic of Moldova, the Russian Federation, Turkey, Turkmenistan and Uzbekistan. Table A2.2 in Annex 2 gives the specific legislation and types of health information required in each country. Several of these countries only introduced legislation in 2018 (i.e. Ireland, Norway, Republic of Moldova and Turkmenistan, plus Member States of the Eurasian Economic Union) and, consequently, it still has to be enacted.

Germany, in 2002, was the first Member State to introduce a regulation covering health information labels on alcopop drinks. France, Germany, Ireland and Lithuania are the only EU Member States with health information legislation (which covers all alcoholic beverages, with the exception of Germany where it is only for alcopops).

Fig. 2. Member States with health information legislation on alcohol labels

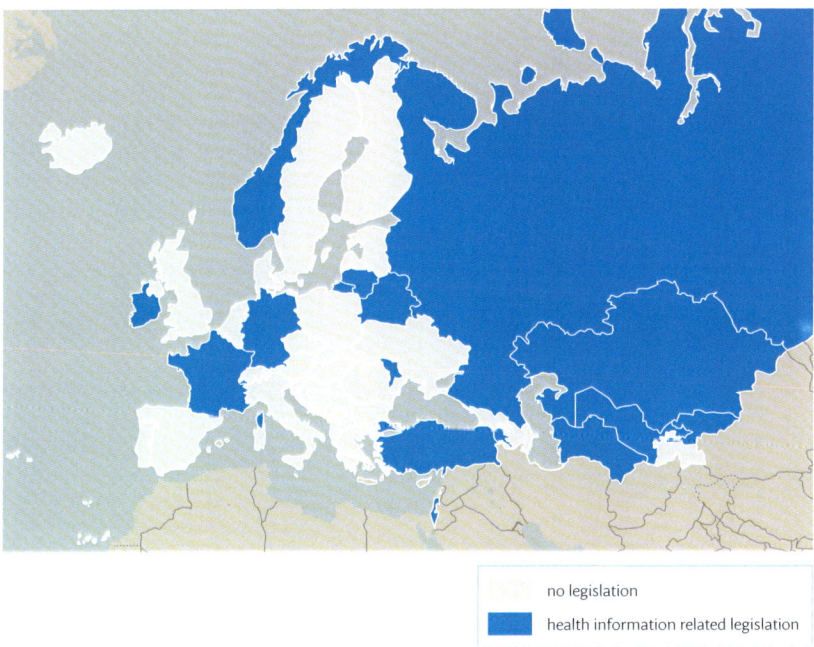

no legislation
health information related legislation

The Eurasian Economic Union introduced a health information regulation obligatory for all its five Member States, mandating inclusion of the message about the dangers of excessive consumption for health on the label of all alcoholic products (Box 2). Some countries (Ireland, Lithuania, Republic of Moldova, the Russian Federation and Turkmenistan) introduced health information labels as part of general national alcohol law, whereas Uzbekistan introduced labelling as part of a joint alcohol and tobacco control law. In other countries, labelling regulations were introduced as part of advertising and marketing restrictions (Israel), protecting young people (Germany) or protecting people with disabilities (France).

While in most cases alcohol labelling messages are mandated to be in written form, there are some countries where the message can also be in pictorial form. For most countries, the decision-making process regarding message content, and whether evidence-informed options were discussed, was unclear. The pictograms used are most commonly the pregnancy logos (France, Lithuania and Republic of Moldova);

Turkey also mandates for pictograms against drinking under 18 years of age and drinking and driving. Unlike for tobacco, no country has yet introduced legislation to use photographs as opposed to symbol/icons.

Size of the message as a minimum percentage of the label is only mandated by law in some countries: no less than 40% of the surface in Uzbekistan, 20% of the surface in Turkmenistan and at least 10% of the surface in the new Eurasian Economic Union regulation. In Turkey, the minimum area and dimension of the message, as well as the type and size of the fonts required, are very precisely specified depending on the size of the product (ranging from 7 cm² total area of the message and font size 6 for products with packaging volume smaller than 100 ml to 30 cm² and font size 12 for products with packaging volume greater than 1000 ml). Similarly, Lithuania mandates the minimum size of the pregnancy logo (5 mm if the volume of the container is 500 ml or less, and 10 mm if the volume exceeds 500 ml). No country uses rotating messages (evidence suggests that changing messages with relative frequency avoids desensitization and keeps the message fresh) or graphic pictorials (photographs) depicting the harm done by alcohol. Table 2 gives an overview of currently used messages in the countries with legislation on health information labelling.

Table 2. Messages specified in health information labelling legislation in the WHO European Region

| Type and topic of message | Message text | Member State |
|---|---|---|
| **Written messages** | | |
| Harm to health | Excessive consumption of alcohol is dangerous to your health | Armenia, Belarus, Kazakhstan, Kyrgyzstan, Russian Federation |
| | Warning: Excessive consumption of alcohol is life threatening and is detrimental to health | Israel |
| | Alcohol is not for children and teenagers up to age 18, pregnant and nursing women, or for persons with diseases of the central nervous system, kidneys, liver, and other digestive organs | Russian Federation |

Table 2 contd

| Type and topic of message | Message text | Member State |
|---|---|---|
| Harm to health (contd) | Alcoholic beverages are harmful to your health! | Turkmenistan |
| | The excessive consumption of alcoholic beverages leads to severe diseases of the human nervous system and internal organs | Uzbekistan |
| Pregnancy | Consumption of alcoholic beverages during pregnancy, even in small amounts, can have serious consequences for the child's health | France |
| Underage | Sale is prohibited to persons under 18 under § 9 of the Youth Protection Act | Germany |
| Other | Warning: Contains alcohol - it is recommended to refrain from excessive consumption | Israel |
| | Alcohol is not your friend | Turkey |
| **Pictograms** | | |
| Driving | 🚫🚗 | Turkey |
| Pregnancy | 🚫🤰 | France, Republic of Moldova, Turkey |
| Underage | ⚠18+ | Turkey |

## 2.2 Industry-led voluntary commitments on labelling for alcoholic beverages

In recent years, there has been an increased number of voluntary actions by the alcohol industry as part of national or international pledges, including specific commitments to the European Alcohol and Health Forum, the European Commission-led stakeholder platform where public and private sectors can pledge actions to tackle harmful levels of alcohol consumption. Sections 2.2.1 and 2.2.2 highlight examples of reporting of voluntary commitments on labelling at European or national levels on ingredients listing, nutritional information or health information. It should be noted that this might not be an exhaustive list of all industry commitments as it reflects the results of the searches carried out for this report.

### 2.2.1 Nutritional labelling

Table A2.3 in Annex 2 summarizes industry commitments related to nutritional information labelling by producers or by producer associations (at the international and national levels). For nutritional labelling, commitments were found particularly from beer producers (95–99), as well as from The Brewers of Europe (100) and some of its national associations (101–104).

At EU level, after the 2017 European Commission labelling report concluding there were no objective grounds that would justify the absence of information on ingredients and nutritional information from alcohol products (68), the industry was given the option to deliver its own proposal for nutritional labelling. In 2018 the European alcoholic beverages sectors submitted a self-regulatory proposal to the European Commission voluntarily providing information on their products, with one common part applicable to the industry as a whole plus separate annexes for beer, spirits, wine, cider and fruit wine sectors (105–109). As the European Commission request referred to listing ingredients and nutritional information only, the proposed information by the industry for the labels included ingredients, energy and nutrient information (energy, total fat, saturated fat, carbohydrates, sugars, protein and salt) per portion size as well as per 100 ml. The proposal allowed this information to be provided either on the label or off-label (e.g. online) and for the information to be presented in a non-standardized way (not aligning with the EU regulation 1169/2011). The Brewers of Europe was the only sector association to commit to including ingredients and nutritional information on labels (106). The Brewers of Europe announced plans to sign a memorandum of understanding with the European Commission in September 2019 to include ingredients and energy values on the labels of all beer bottles and cans in the EU by the end of 2022 (110). The other sectors (spirits, wine, cider and fruit wine sectors) did not fully commit to include the ingredients and nutritional information on the label and, instead, stayed with the option of providing the information online (105,107,109). In June 2019 spiritsEUROPE signed a memorandum of understanding with the European Commission committing to providing energy values on the label but the other information online (ingredients and full nutritional values) (111).

While many of the commitments, particularly from the beer sector, reflect the recommendations in the WHO discussion paper on policy options for alcohol labelling by including both ingredients and a full list of nutritional values on the label, some of the commitments are worded in such a way as to allow information to be published online rather than on the label.

### 2.2.2 Health information labelling

Table A2.3 in Annex 2 presents the commitments for health information labelling made by producers and associations. In 2013 the world's biggest beer, wine and spirits producers made a series of joint commitments to reduce the harmful use of alcohol (112). The labelling-related commitment included health information labelling as follows: provide consumer information through the products carrying symbols or words warning against harmful drinking of their products worldwide.

Health information labelling commitments could be identified for individual producers (97,113–117). Some of these preceded the joint commitments, with some pledged at national level (Greece, the Netherlands, Portugal, Spain, Sweden and the United Kingdom) (118–127). In general, commitments most commonly referred to inclusion of "pictograms related to pregnancy, underage drinking and drinking and driving". While industry has committed to putting some health information on labels, so far this has been mainly limited to inclusion of pictograms and has not specified precise size and visibility as called for by the WHO discussion paper on policy options for alcohol labelling (62).

## 2.3 Monitoring implementation of alcohol labelling

Independent monitoring is essential to understand the level of implementation of alcohol labelling. This section summarizes the very few reports found on the implementation of industry commitments and the single independent monitoring study at EU level. No studies were identified for national legislation implementation or for non-EU WHO European Region Member States.

### 2.3.1 Evidence from independent monitoring at EU level

A major EU study commissioned by the Executive Agency for Health and Consumers on behalf of the European Commission audited labelling implemented in practice by monitoring the presence of health and nutritional information on labels of alcoholic drinks in supermarkets in 15 EU Member States (Belgium, Czechia,

Denmark, France, Germany, Greece, Ireland, Italy, Latvia, the Netherlands, Poland, Portugal, Romania, Spain and the United Kingdom) during the summer months of 2013 (129). This is the only cross-national study identifying what is included and present on the labels of alcoholic drinks available to customers from premises in those countries.

From the audited countries (Fig. 3), only France and Germany had legislative mandates to include health information in the labels. France, the only country with mandated labelling to include a pregnancy warning, showed 100% compliance, whereas Germany, with government-mandated labelling to include an age limit message, showed low compliance (8.4%). Labelling activities in the other instances were the result of industry voluntary action or pledges (at national or EU levels, as the results combine the domestic and imported product). In the countries without

Fig. 3. Health and nutritional information given on alcohol labels, by country

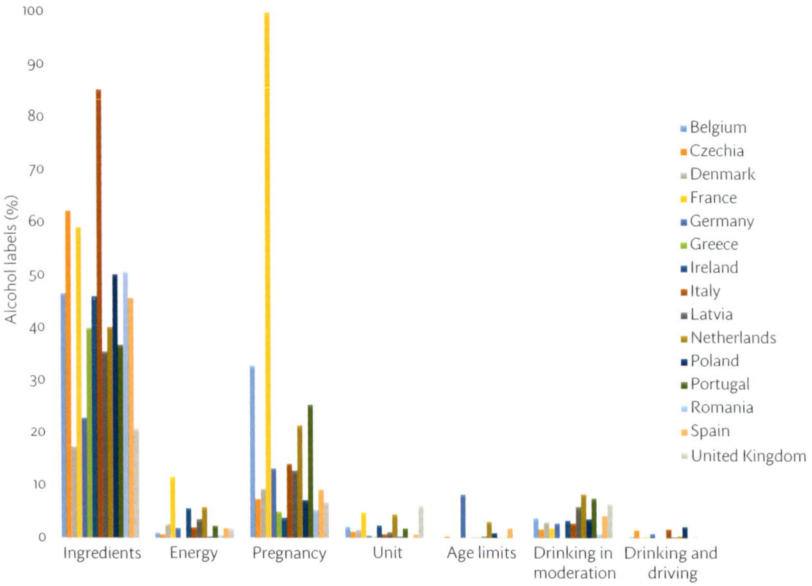

Source: based on data in Botterman et al., 2014 (129).

any regulations mandating labelling, the percentages of presence of information were very low, apart from information on ingredients and pregnancy warnings. Across all 15 audited Member States, 17% of labels carried a least one of the audited health messages (4374 beverage packages). The percentage was highest in France, where the pregnancy logo was obligatory (100%), followed by Belgium (35%), Portugal (30%) and the Netherlands (29%), and lowest in Greece and Ireland (both 5%).

In total, 25 730 beverage packages (approximately 50% for wines, 25% for beer and 25% for spirits) were audited for the presence of five different health messages from four retailers of differing sizes in each of the 15 countries. Warnings for pregnant women were by far the most common, with other messages being shown in much smaller percentages. The messages were most common on wine bottles (19%) and less frequently found on spirits (13%) and beers (11%) (Table 3).

Information on nutrition on the label was assessed for the 4374 products with at least one health message on the packaging. Information on sulphites was present on almost all beers and spirits that also carried a health message, and on over half of wines. From the same sample, while 82% of beers, 32% of wines and 39% of spirits contained a list of ingredients, information on calories was present only on 6% of beer products, 1% of wines and 3% of spirits (129).

### 2.3.2 Evidence from industry-led voluntary commitments

There is no formal mechanism established in any part of the Region or at country level to audit or keep track of voluntary commitments on alcohol labelling, with most being self-reported. Generally, there is also a lack of literature evaluating the implementation of voluntary commitments (130), either from independent research or from industry bodies. With a few exceptions (e.g. some specific commitments to the European Alcohol and Health Forum), little could be found on whether, or how, these commitments were implemented, monitored and evaluated. Where reports on compliance with commitments were identified, details of the methodology used was often lacking.

At company level, information was only found for Carlsberg (132) and Heineken (131) on the percentage of products containing nutritional information (Table A2.3 in Annex 2), with Heineken reporting that 95% of its beers and ciders worldwide had nutritional information in 2018 (on pack or online), and Carlsberg reporting that

Table 3: Message types present on different alcohol products

| Drink type | Warning for pregnant women (%) | Information about units/grams (%) | Legal age limit for purchasing or consuming alcoholic beverages (%) | Messages about drinking in moderation (%) | Drinking and driving (%) |
|---|---|---|---|---|---|
| Beer | 11.4 | 2.5 | 1.5 | 4.5 | 2.3 |
| Wine | 18.7 | 1.7 | 0.0 | 1.8 | 0.1 |
| Spirit | 13.4 | 0.9 | 1.7 | 4.5 | 0.1 |
| Other (cider, alcopops, etc.) | 7.8 | 4.5 | 1.1 | 6.9 | 0.1 |
| Overall | 17.0 | 2.0 | 1.0 | 3.0 | 1.0 |

*Note:* audit of 25 730 alcoholic beverages in 15 EU Member States.
*Source:* data derived from Botterman et al., 2014 (129).

65% of its total beer volume listed nutritional information and 85% listed ingredient information. In both cases, the data were provided as part of an annual report that was reviewed by external independent auditors, but no clear information was provided on the method for deriving these figures. Similarly, The Brewers of Europe provided percentages for their overall commitment (133) and reported that 85% and 60% of the pre-packaged beers in the EU in 2019 carried labels for ingredients and calories, respectively. However, again, no background methodology on how those numbers were obtained was provided.

Some companies reported compliance of 96–100% with their own health information commitments (113,117,132,134,135). Based on the self-report from the Beer, Wine and Spirit Producers' Commitments (a collaboration of the world's leading beer, wine and spirit companies), health information messages in 2017 were present on 85% of products of companies reporting by volume and on 59% of products of companies reporting by brands (112). However, in most cases, no detailed methods for deriving these percentages were available in the reports, with the exception of one economic operator (135). While it is common that external auditors review the results of self-monitoring, in the case of the Producers' Commitments, the key performance indicator for health information labelling was not one of those reviewed (112).

At country level, the Netherlands is a good example of scaling up of the labelling commitment, as self-reporting from the Foundation for Responsible Alcohol Consumption highlighted an increase of health information labelling over the course of three years: on beer products, from 0.5% in 2013 to 99.6% in 2016; on wine products, from 46% to 81%; and on spirits, from 31% to 71% (121). No information was available on how the evaluation was carried out, on the characteristics of the logo itself (e.g. size, visibility), on any effects on awareness and of any plans to continue monitoring in the future. In the United Kingdom, self-regulation under the Public Health Responsibility Deal of 2013 has witnessed the development and evaluation of the alcoholic beverage producers' pledge to include health information on their product labels (Case study 1) (128). No other monitoring or self-reporting information could be identified for national voluntary commitments in other countries.

### Case study 1. Voluntary commitments and self-regulation in the United Kingdom

The United Kingdom has witnessed a long-standing debate on the merits of a voluntary versus a mandatory approach. Health information labelling was first discussed in 1991, with the first agreement between the United Kingdom Government and the alcohol industry to include alcohol unit content on labels in 1998 *(136)*. In 2003 there was a proposal to introduce tobacco-style warnings on all alcoholic products, along with recommendations on low-risk drinking limits *(69)*. However, the United Kingdom Government decided to pursue an industry-led self-regulatory path and established a voluntary agreement with the alcohol industry in 2007 *(137)*.

#### Voluntary agreement

The voluntary agreement on alcohol labelling included the following: unit alcohol content in the container, warning about drinking alcohol in pregnancy (either as text or pictogram) and signposting to the Drinkaware website (www.drinkaware.co.uk; an industry-funded alcohol awareness charity). There was also a set of optional recommendations: the low-risk weekly drinking guidelines message ("The United Kingdom Chief Medical Officers recommend adults do not regularly drink more than 14 units per week"), calorie content, drinking and driving message (e.g. "don't drink and drive" logo), responsibility statement ("Drink Responsibly", "Enjoy Responsibly", "Drink in Moderation", "Drink Sensibly" or "Know your Limits") and age-restricted product (by logo) *(137)*.

Evaluation studies showed that the commitments were largely not met *(138–140)*; in the 2009 assessment, only 8% of the sample was content compliant with all five requirements present *(140)*.

#### Strengthening labelling implementation

The United Kingdom Government then launched a consultation with three options: to continue with the current agreement, to strengthen the current agreement (based on suggestions from the industry) or to introduce mandatory labelling *(70)*. The consultation highlighted a major difference in opinion, with almost all non-industry stakeholders supporting a mandatory labelling scheme and almost all industry-related stakeholders opposing it. The industry suggested strengthened self-regulation was feasible, with the Portman Group (an industry membership body) supporting this scheme by helping

### Case study 1 contd

its implementation. The United Kingdom Government decided to go with the second consultation option – to strengthen the current self-regulation agreement (136).

In 2011 an extended voluntary labelling scheme with the same elements was introduced as part of the Public Health Responsibility Deal, where the alcohol producers could commit to ensure that 80% their products would contain three required elements (units, low-risk guidelines and pregnancy warning) on the label by the end of 2013 (138,141). The Portman Group took responsibility for issuing voluntary guidelines, and additionally issued best practice guidance (142). In 2016 the United Kingdom Chief Medical Officers (CMOs) changed the official low-risk drinking guidelines to a maximum of 14 units per week for women and men (142). The Portman Group guidance was revised in 2017 (128) and it was no longer recommended that the message on low-risk drinking guidelines should be placed on the product label. However, in 2019 the Portman Group announced that it was encouraging all drink producers to include the low-risk guidelines on their labels (143).

### Effectiveness

Results of an independent evaluation of the Public Health Responsibility Deal pledge in 2014 showed that 77% of all 156 surveyed products contained three of the five required elements and 72% contained all five elements (71). The researchers concluded that the labelling pledge with regard to unit content and health information label was not fully met, particularly in aspects related to clarity. For example, the mean font size used for products with guidelines was 8.17 point, while font size 10–11 was considered optimal for legibility. In terms of size and colouring of the pregnancy health information logo, the mean size was 5.95 mm and the most common colour was grey (71).

In 2017 the Alcohol Health Alliance UK published the results of another audit of compliance of alcohol labels with the new CMO drinking guidelines. Out of 315 products reviewed, only one product informed customers of the new weekly guideline of 14 units. When the products referred to unit limits in the United Kingdom, they referred to old guidelines. No products advised consumers to spread their drinking across three or more days or to have drink-free days, and there were no health information labels. Almost all of the reviewed products, however, included the pregnancy warning (144). A further report from

### Case study 1 contd

the Alcohol Health Alliance UK with data from 2018 showed that 284 out of 320 reviewed products (89%) included the pregnancy logo, but many were small and difficult to see. While 24 (8%) included the new CMO guidelines, 211 (66%) referred to out-of-date limits (145). Another study in the United Kingdom in 2017 examined 156 products for calorie information on the labels and found only two (1.3%) carrying such information (72).

### Next steps

The industry was set a deadline of September 2019 to update product labels to state accurately the new CMO low-risk guidelines, and the Scottish Government's 2018 alcohol strategy confirmed that it will consider mandating health information labelling if producers do not meet the deadline (146).

## 2.4 Alignment of labelling practices with WHO recommendations

The WHO discussion paper on policy options for alcohol labelling (62) made a number of recommendations and this section assesses national legislation and industry commitments for alignment with these recommendations.

### 2.4.1 National legislation

Looking at what nutritional information is required by existing regulations in Member States of the WHO European Region (Table A2.1 in Annex 2), there is a tendency for labelling regulations to mandate information on ingredients (40% of Member States) as opposed to information on nutritional values (19% of Member States, with all of these also including ingredients listing). Only 10 out of the 53 Member States (19%) have legislation that includes both, thus aligning in full with the WHO policy recommendations for alcohol labelling.

Considering the recommendations for health information in the WHO discussion paper on policy options for alcohol labelling (62), 15 of the 53 WHO European Region Member States (28%) have introduced some legislation to include health-related information on the label; yet in only nine countries (17%) does the legislation specify the size of the message, and only seven of those specify a minimum percentage of the label to be used (ranging from 10% to 40%). Five Member States have some specifications on format of the text. No legislation mentions rotating messages or informational images.

### 2.4.2 Industry commitments

In terms of nutritional information labelling, some of the industry commitments (particularly for beers) refer to alignment of their product labelling with the general EU regulation and so would be in line with the WHO recommendations. Based on self-reported data from The Brewers of Europe, 85% of pre-packaged beers in the EU label ingredients and 60% label calories. However, most of the producers and producers' associations, particularly in the wine and spirits sectors, are in favour of providing the nutritional information online rather than on the label, which makes the commitments less straightforward and not in line with the recommendation for provision of information on labels.

In terms of health information labelling, some producers have committed to introduce pictograms encouraging consumers not to drink and drive and not to drink while pregnant or if underage. Based on self-report, health information messages were present on 85% of products of the major companies reporting by volume and on 59% of products of those reporting by brands (112). In most cases, the commitment focused only on the presence of the message on the label and no specifications were made on how the message should be presented (what should be its size or how to ensure its visibility) and so again did not align with the WHO recommendations.

## 2.5 Factors supporting the development and implementation of regulatory frameworks for alcohol labelling

Based on the reviewed evidence, the main themes emerged as either facilitating or hindering factors when developing and implementing labelling regulations, although some factors had both facilitating and hindering features (e.g. consumer pressures). These are presented in this section (supportive factors) and section 2.6 (hindering factors), along with specific country examples.

### 2.5.1 Labels introduced as part of a larger package of alcohol control measures

When alcohol labelling has been successfully introduced in regulation, it has normally been as part of a larger package of measures aimed at curbing alcohol-related harm, either produced at the same time or in close succession. This has eased the introduction of labelling itself and, overall, has resulted in stronger policy packages that are more effective in reducing alcohol-related harm (147).

For example, in Israel, the introduction of health information labels on alcohol products in 2014 was part of a broader law aimed at limiting the advertising and marketing of alcoholic products. The other measures in the bill included a ban on outdoor advertising, print items and television advertisements directed at children and adolescents; a ban on the use of alcohol products as gifts, giveaways or prizes; limitation on the appearance, structure and quantity of advertisements, both in print and on the Internet; and requirement for a warning notice on the permitted advertisements. Ingredients and nutritional listings were not identified specifically in the package of measures included in the law. Additionally, at that point, reform in the taxation of alcoholic products was also being implemented that aimed to increase the price of low-cost, high-alcohol items (138).

In Lithuania, following the mandatory legislation for ingredients listing, the 2016 law introducing the obligatory graphic warnings about the alcohol harm for pregnant women was also part of a more comprehensive alcohol control policy, which within a short period of time introduced several measures: lowering the legal blood alcohol content limit to 0.00 for novice, professional and motorbike drivers; forbidding the selling of alcohol at petrol stations; and increasing excise tax (148). This was followed by even stricter measures in 2018: a total ban on alcohol advertising, an increase to 20 years as the legal age to buy alcohol and shorter selling hours (149).

In Ireland, the alcohol labelling legislation introduced in 2018 as a part of Public Health (Alcohol) Act, mandating inclusion of both health information and energy content, was part of a comprehensive alcohol policy package, which also included mandating minimum price per gram of alcohol, restricting advertising of alcohol products, and physically separating alcohol products in retail outlets (83).

In 2006 the Russian Federation introduced a package of measures to curb unrecorded consumption (due to high rates of production in the informal sector), including the introduction of labelling for non-beverage alcohol. Amendments to the Federal Law No. 171 were made in December 2006 (150) and the newly added paragraph stated:

> Apart from other compulsory details, the labels of alcohol-containing non-food productsintended for retail sale shall contain information about the danger for human life or health of the use of such products for food

purposes (in this case the word "denatured" shall be used in place of the words "ethyl alcohol" when reference is made to denatured alcohol-containing products). This information shall be located on the front side of the label and it shall occupy at least 10 per cent of the area thereof (except for labels for perfume and cosmetics products).

Overall, evidence also points to the effectiveness of supplementing labelling with an integrated evidence-informed strategy that, in addition to point-of-purchase information, advertisements, and package inserts, includes broader communication actions, such as those aimed at changing social norms (151).

### 2.5.2 Strong political support for introduction of the legislation

Strong political will has played a role in pushing forward alcohol control policies, including labelling. Recognition of the direct and indirect harm done by alcohol and the associated costs of alcohol consumption has contributed to making this issue a political priority.

For example, historically, Ireland had no systematic approach to alcohol policy. In 2009 alcohol was first included in a National Substance Misuse Strategy, followed by a 2012 Steering Group Report on a National Substance Misuse Strategy (192). The Report included 45 recommendations to integrate alcohol policy into the National Substance Misuse Strategy across supply, prevention, treatment, rehabilitation and research. Based on the Report and reflecting the so-called best buys from WHO global and European strategies, the main measures to be included in the Public Health (Alcohol) Bill (minimum unit pricing, labelling of alcoholic products and restrictions on alcohol marketing) were then agreed by the Irish Government in 2013 with the intention of drafting and enacting the Bill swiftly (152). (However, opposition from other EU Member States and the alcohol industry delayed advancing the Bill; see sections 2.5.1 and 2.5.2.) Reasons for this strong approach to policy in 2013 were related to high alcohol consumption, high rates of binge drinking and consequently a high prevalence of alcohol problems in Ireland (153).

In Lithuania, which used to have one of the highest rates of alcohol consumption in the WHO European Region, the societal and political climate was favourable to alcohol control in 2016 when the regulation was passed. Parliament received proposals regarding alcohol regulations, one of which was backed with 60 000 signatures from civil society and supported by a leading political party. The party that came to power in October 2016 had advocated tackling alcohol harm in the country as one of its main campaign promises; consequently, many new representatives in the Parliament had promised stricter alcohol control. The Prime Minister and Minister of Health both came from the newly elected party, which further facilitated the changes (148).

### 2.5.3 Consumer pressure

The views of consumers and pressure from consumer groups have played a strong role both in facilitating and in hindering the development of alcohol legislation, including alcohol labelling. For example, warnings regarding drinking alcohol during pregnancy in France were first proposed in 2004 as an amendment to the law on disabled people's rights (154). Initially, the amendment was rejected; however, after a lawsuit threat by three mothers of children with fetal alcohol syndrome for not informing them about the dangers of drinking alcohol during pregnancy, and the accompanying press attention, the Government proposed legislation (Case study 2) (73,155).

Case study 2. Mandatory labelling implementation in France

In 2005 France introduced a law mandating labelling for all alcoholic beverages that warned against drinking during pregnancy.

Implementation

In the legal draft, a health message mentioning "the dangers of excessive consumption of alcohol and recommending abstinence for pregnant women" was planned; however, in the final version, the alcohol industry was allowed to choose between a written message and a pictogram, which led to most producers using the pictogram (73). Because of strong lobbying by the alcohol industry, minimal specification regarding the size and colour of the pictogram were established, which resulted in the use of a small pictogram (4 mm in diameter) with low visibility (156).

The implementation of the pregnancy warning was embedded in the wider strategy to raise awareness of the potential harms of drinking alcohol during pregnancy (157). There was an accompanying communication campaign in print media and radio, with the main message "Zero alcohol during pregnancy". The message was also displayed in the pregnancy notebook sent to every French pregnant woman and was distributed on flyers to health facilities

## Case study 2 contd

providing care for pregnant women (73,158). Additionally, both epidemiological monitoring and improved training for health professionals were implemented to supplement the campaign (157).

### Effectiveness

There have been some efforts to measure the effectiveness of the warning label and the surrounding campaign. One study examined changes in knowledge and social norms regarding drinking in pregnancy by comparing phone surveys made in 2004 and in 2007 (159). This indicated a slight improvement in awareness in 2007 compared with 2004 of the recommendation that pregnant women should not drink (87% vs 82%). In the 2015 follow-up study, 84% of respondents answered that pregnant women should not drink alcohol and 72% thought it was not advised to drink beer while breastfeeding (193). A more recent cross-sectional survey with a large representative sample of women who were either pregnant or had just given birth (158) found that the warning label had been noticed by 66% of women overall and by 77% of women who drank. Almost all women who noticed the label thought it suggested abstinence. However, 41% of the women mistakenly thought spirits were more harmful than wine or beer (158). Additionally, qualitative analysis of the pictogram's effectiveness showed that the warning suffered from lack of visibility because of its size, and the pictograms were considered as "weak and insufficient" by the participants (74).

Evaluation of the French law and its implementation underline the importance of size and position of the warnings, echoing recommendations in the WHO discussion paper on policy options for alcohol labelling, and the need to ensure that complementary information is in place in order that the risks of alcohol, the meaning of standard drinks and the associated harm across alcohol categories are understood (158).

### Next steps

Currently, the French Health Minister has introduced in the National Public Health Plan 2018–2022 (194), a measure to improve the visibility of the pregnancy logo; this measure is present also in the French National Plan for Mobilization Against Addictions 2018–2022 (160).

### 2.5.4 A stepwise incremental process

The country examples documented in this report show that not all legislation is introduced in a single step. In some cases, a less comprehensive law or smaller package of measures is agreed and passed as a first step to further revisions. Dividing the process into smaller requests facilitates achieving a full labelling policy eventually. For example, in the Russian Federation, Federal Law No. 171 (which also regulates alcohol labelling) was introduced in 1995 (150) but has since been amended more than 40 times (Case study 3). Dividing changes into smaller requests facilitates the process of achieving the full labelling policy in line with WHO recommendations.

#### Case study 3. Stepwise changes in legislation in the Russian Federation

The 2007 Alcohol Law of the Russian Federation included Decree No. 49, which was issued by the Ministry of Health and Social Development of the Russian Federation and approved warning labels on consumer packaging of products regarding the contraindications for alcoholic beverage use (161). The Decree introduced mandatory health information with the following wording: "Alcohol is contraindicated in children and adolescents under 18, pregnant and lactating women, persons with diseases of the central nervous system, kidneys, liver and other digestive organs". However, beer and related alcoholic beverages based on it were not officially recognized as alcoholic beverages at that point and several separate regulations for beer existed, with no mandatory health information labelling. The July 2011 amendments to the Federal Law No. 171 officially changed the status of beer to an alcoholic beverage, even if the changes did not come into force until 2013. The amendments of July 2011 also made additional information on alcohol volume mandatory (in 100 ml of the product as well as in the entire volume of the container) and required more extensive health hazards warnings in addition to those already present in the regulation on health information labels from 2007.

## 2.6 Factors hindering the development and implementation of regulatory frameworks for alcohol labelling

### 2.6.1 Opposition from international organizations and their members

When proposing labelling legislation, the proponent country has in some cases had to respond to opposition from other European countries after they were notified of the proposed legislation. Such criticism and opposition are mainly issued through larger transnational institutions.

In Ireland, the Bill including regulation on alcohol labelling was published in 2015 (152). As a member of the EU, Ireland was required to take part in the EU notification procedure.[2] During the process, the Irish Government received a private warning from the European Commission (162) and had to respond to comments from seven EU Member States (Denmark, France, Greece, Romania, Slovakia, Spain and the United Kingdom) and detailed opinions from further two Member States (Italy and Portugal) (163). This resulted in a consultation process that only closed on 20 April 2018 and was then extended to 20 July 2018, which delayed the process of advancing the Bill. Some of the comments, for example, were from countries with large wine-producing industries that were concerned about the prospect of cancer warnings on drink labels (164).

In Finland, a proposal was discussed in 2007 for a law that would mandate for alcohol products to carry a health information label "WARNING: Alcohol endangers foetal development and your health" (165,166). However, the law was repealed in 2008 before it came into force (101,102). Reasons for abolishing the proposed warning labels included, in particular, opposition from the EU (the European Commission provided a negative opinion during the notification procedure), as well as opposition from the Finnish alcohol industry and a change of government policy (101,102).

A recent analysis of the minutes of the World Trade Organization's Committee on Technical Barriers to Trade meetings from 2010 to 2018 examined notifications about alcohol labelling proposals (which included ones from Ireland, Israel and Turkey) (21). The Organization's 164 Member States were most concerned with the content of the warning messages, use of emotive and realistic imagery as part of the messages, mandatory requirements for message design and placement, prescribed rotation of the warnings, prohibition of stickers or supplementary labels, and restriction of the industry's choice of words and images for the beverage label (21). For example, the EU was opposing Israel's requirement to have the health information label on the front of the pack with the argument that it would be burdensome and costly for imports (21). The Turkish original proposal had very strict requirements on the

---

2. The (EU) 2015/1535 notification procedure is intended to prevent the creation of barriers in the internal market before they materialize. Member States notify their legislative projects regarding products and these are analysed by the European Commission in the light of EU legislation. Member States participate equally with the Commission in this procedure and they can also issue their opinions on the notified drafts.

layout and design of the label, which was again criticized by the EU as excessive. In both cases, the proposals were later amended to be less restrictive.

### 2.6.2 Opposition and lobbying from the alcohol industry

The alcohol industry has been described as being very active in conveying its views at Member State or EU Parliament level (75). In the United Kingdom, for example, the industry is seen as participating fully in Government consultations, where their representatives advocate against effective policies that would reduce their profit, such as minimum alcohol pricing and other price interventions (167). An evidence review by Public Health England of the alcohol control policies in the United Kingdom in 2017 suggested that the producer-led actions have not had a favourable impact on public health (195).

In Ireland, the enactment of the Public Health (Alcohol) Bill of 2015 was delayed for almost three years, with opposition from the alcohol industry being considered one of the principal reasons, although not the only one, for such a long delay (168). During the parliamentary passage of the Bill, lobbying from the alcohol industry increased both directly with members of Irish legislature (169) and through campaigning against the proposed Bill (168). Some of the arguments against the proposed legislative programme were the negative effects of the Bill on the Irish economy and the alcohol industry (particularly for the small producers) (170), along with predictions of job losses (168) and decrease of export ability because of the labelling requirements (171). In an assessment of the socioeconomic impacts of the proposed regulations under the Bill commissioned by the industry, the main impacts of labelling on the consumer put forward were reduced choice and increased prices of products (through rising production costs and reduced competition) (170). Additionally, the relative size of the health information labels was questioned (170). Personal autonomy and increased education, mostly ineffective measures on their own, were suggested by the industry as suitable alternatives to legislation (168). Further discourse analysis pointed out that industry communications framed the issue as pertaining to personal responsibility and considered alcohol as an economic commodity rather than a harmful substance (172).

In France, the draft plans of the Minister for Health proposing to increase the size of the pregnancy logo and move it to the front of the bottle, as well as to introduce a health information label about alcohol not being suitable for those under 18 years of age (173), were met with strong opposition by a group of leading wine producers in the country (173). This resulted in a slight modification of the plans, with only the inclusion of a measure to improve the visibility of the pregnancy logo in the National Public Health Plan 2018–2022 (194).

In some parts of the Region, the alcohol industry is very active in influencing discussions around the regulation of alcohol products (75). In 2007 the EU almost introduced regulations mandating health information labels on alcoholic drinks, but this clause was removed as a result of industry lobbying (75). Regulation 1169/2011 on the provision of food information to consumers (63) covers all foods and soft drink products but for alcoholic beverages only has mandatory requirements for information on the most common allergens in alcoholic beverages (e.g. sulphites added to wine) and the alcoholic strength by volume for beverages containing more than 1.2% alcohol by volume. In 2017 the European Commission labelling report concluded that there were no objective grounds that would justify the absence of information on ingredients and nutritional information from alcohol products (68) but the industry was given the option of delivering its own proposals (Box 3). Tactics used to influence discussions include controlling the public health debate and setting an agenda that reflects the industry's priorities (e.g. promoting actions with less public health impact and never including regulation) (75). This influence is achieved also by participating in meetings and panels, through corporate responsibility activities and through involvement in social organizations/events, such as the European Parliament Beer Club and Annual Cocktail Party (75).

---

Box 3. Industry responses to nutritional information provision in the EU

In response to the 2017 European Commission labelling report (section 2.2.1) (68), the alcoholic beverage industry was given a year to prepare a self-regulatory proposal covering the whole sector of alcoholic beverages.

The self-regulatory proposals put forward in 2018 (105–109) had one part applicable to the industry as a whole and a second series of annexes for beer, spirits, wine and the cider and fruit wine sectors). The proposal covered ingredients, energy and nutrient information on a portion size as well as for 100 ml but it did not specify that this information had to be provided on the label (i.e. leaving the option of online provision) nor on a standardized method for the presentation of information (i.e. to align with EU Regulation 1169/2011). The push for off-label provision of information was criticized by the EU's health commissioner (185) for inconsistency, by some Members of European Parliament (186) and by civil society organizations (187).

In 2019 it was under assessment by the European Commission, which would then go into another impact assessment phase to review further options, both regulatory and non-regulatory. In 2019 the only developments had been the

> Box 3 contd
>
> beer and spirits sectors signing a memorandum of understanding on including the ingredients and energy values: The Brewers of Europe opted for doing so completely on labels and spiritsEUROPE for doing so partly on labels (110,111).

Similar to the tobacco industry, the alcohol industry, with the support of governments in alcohol-exporting nations, has looked to international trade and investment law as a means of opposing health information labels on alcohol (175,176). Legal arguments and claims against alcohol control policies have been used in Iceland and the European Economic Area, for example to attack the introduction of alcohol marketing restrictions such as banning or limiting the visual imagery of the packaging of alcoholic beverages and making their contents more salient through mandatory labelling (175).

Similar instances have occurred worldwide. For example, for pregnancy warnings, the most commonly agreed labelling practice, the alcohol industry in Australia has lobbied to undermine community concern; debated the evidence for labelling by suggesting that mandatory alcohol warning labels could have adverse effects for pregnant women, including prompting the unnecessary termination of pregnancies; and questioned the efficacy of alcohol warning labels (174). In Yukon Territory, in Canada, the alcohol industry raised a "large range of legal concerns" and succeeded in removing new labels from bottles and cans warning that "Alcohol can cause cancer, including breast and colon cancers", which had been experimentally introduced to test their effects (176). The raising of legal doubts, threats of litigation and the actual commencement of litigation have worked for tobacco-related issues and have the potential to deter governments from implementing health information labelling for alcohol (177).

### 2.6.3 Legislative processes at country level slowed down by international procedures

Member States of the EU must inform the European Commission of any draft technical regulation prior to its adoption to ensure that other Member States can give their opinions on issues that might create barriers to the free movement of goods (see section 2.6.1, which discusses the notification procedure). A Member State has to wait for three months for the response from the European Commission or other Member States and then respond to comments, leading to a further three-month delay. The Commission can block the draft for 12–18 months if EU harmonization work is being undertaken in the same field (178). This process delayed the process of confirming legislation in Ireland (section 2.6.1); it took three years of debate and responses to opponents, at both the EU and national levels, before the bill was passed and signed into law by the President on 17 October 2018. After the bill was enacted, the regulation on the introduction of labels still had to be notified to the EU before its commencement can apply, with a three-year transition period after the start of the implementation (179).

Legislative processes at country level have also been slowed through waiting for the EU's next steps in terms of suggested regulation on alcohol labelling. In Norway, for example, the Parliament voted to include health labelling on alcohol products in 2015 (180). Despite labelling being mentioned in national alcohol strategies for almost a decade and rallying general support from many parties, the proposal did not succeed as the majority wanted to first see the outcome of the EU process on the issue (180). Delays in the EU process have led to delays in action at national level. A similar situation has occurred in Austria (181), where it was decided that the country would comply if the EU decided to regulate health information labelling, but this would not be initiated on a national basis.

In the Russian Federation, the Ministry of Health announced in August 2018 that it was reviewing a new initiative on graphical health information labels for alcoholic beverages that would show images of the consequences of harmful alcohol use, as done with tobacco. The measure was suggested by a group of parliamentarians and the Ministry explored ways of including the suggested measures into the national Strategy for the Formation of a Healthy Lifestyle for the Population until 2025 (182) but no specific images were determined. In December 2018 the initiative was rejected because it also proposed certain other measures that were not considered feasible (183). However, the Ministry emphasized the need for health information labelling and pointed out that this measure cannot be carried out in the Russian Federation alone because of the need to comply with the technical regulations of the Eurasian Economic Union. The Federal Antimonopoly Service of the Russian Federation also announced in December 2018 that it was in favour of unified health information labels on alcoholic beverages with the slogan "Alcohol kills", as proposed by the group of parliamentarians (184).

### 2.6.4 Economic and cultural arguments opposing the introduction of alcohol labelling

Opposition to the introduction of alcohol labelling legislation often uses arguments related to the negative effects of labelling on the economy. In France, for example, during the debate on the introduction of pregnancy warnings, the arguments against the amendment predominantly focused on political, cultural and economic factors (158). In Ireland, arguments against the proposed legislative programme included the negative effects of the bill on the Irish economy and on the alcohol industry, as well as predictions of job and export losses (168). The argument (mostly led by wine producers) that drinking is intrinsic to the culture in some European countries and part of the daily culture, and that most consumers drink in moderation, has equally been used as a strong lobby against labelling practices and to slow down discussions on alcohol labelling (188,189).

### 2.6.5 Lack of precise specifications for message appearance on the label

When a regulation on the presence of a message on labels is passed but there are no specifications on design of the label, producers are likely to find a way of implementing the message to cause as little visual disturbance in the product as possible. This was the situation in France (156), where minimal regulation on the size of the logo were put forward in the regulations, resulting in the pregnancy warnings being barely visible (156). In Turkey, the law gave precise specifications, in line with the suggestions in the WHO document on policy options on alcohol labelling (62), with the displayed warning having three pictograms (against drinking under 18 years of age, drinking and driving, and drinking in pregnancy) and the text "Alcohol is not your friend" (190). The exact size of the message and the fonts for different sizes of containers, as well as other aspects of the label (visibility, colour), were also specified in the text of the law (190).

### 2.6.6 Lack of monitoring and enforcement of initiatives

Establishing rules but not monitoring and enforcing them will very likely lead to a poor outcome. In the United Kingdom, which has voluntary commitments, the Portman Group is responsible for issuing the best practice guidelines but no official authority is designated to monitor and enforce the agreement (138). Several audits have been published showing that the pledge has not been implemented according to the agreement (Case study 1) (139,140), but there is no evidence of the imposition of sanctions.

There are few monitoring initiatives for the enforcement of labelling (mandated or voluntary) in the WHO European Region, making it difficult to assess the implementation fidelity and penetration of existing agreements. When it comes to industry self-monitoring, the available monitoring reports (112,117,131,132) reveal some common points: the focus has been primarily on presenting the results, with less emphasis on describing the methodology and its potential shortcomings. These results are often in company reports and are checked by external independent auditors, who confirm whether the report has been prepared in accordance with criteria the companies have set out for themselves in a limited audit. A more rigorous scientific approach, for example that used in the independent evaluation of the United Kingdom's Public Health Responsibility Deal (71), would be preferable as it would provide more transparent and objective information on industry compliance with its own commitments.

# 3. DISCUSSION

## 3.1 Strengths and limitations of this review

This review is unique in that it presents a comprehensive picture on what is the current alcohol labelling practice in the WHO European Region (2019), either through regulations or through voluntary commitments from the industry, and it gives examples of establishment of national regulations, and implementation success factors in various countries. Previous reports have focused either on presenting an overview of regulations, mainly in the EU (65–67), or of suggested labelling practices. No review to date has compiled experiences and analysed lessons learned from countries on introducing alcohol labelling practice through legislation or voluntary commitments. The review includes a comprehensive grey literature analysis in addition to the systematic review of the academic literature, as such policy-related topics are not commonly found in peer-reviewed journals.

### 3.1.1 Lack of peer-reviewed literature

Only a small number of peer-reviewed articles could be identified that described the presence of alcohol labelling, its implementation or the evaluation of existing policies in the WHO European Region. These could not be assessed for quality as they were mainly descriptive in nature. This may reflect the difficulties outlined in the Results of actual implementation as well as the fact that only nine Member States in the Region include both nutritional and health information on alcoholic beverage labelling. Even when labelling has been implemented, there were few studies evaluating the implementation process or its impact. There is even less literature on the effects of specific messages (e.g. cancer warnings) in real-life settings. This is partly because attempts to carry out larger-scale experiments on labelling with different warnings have been stopped by industry in several instances (e.g. the study in the Yukon Territory (176)).

### 3.1.2 Myriad of European languages

A strength of this review is the lack of restrictions on publication language and date for the peer-reviewed literature and the few language restrictions for grey literature. This ensured a comprehensive search of both peer-reviewed and grey literature, including government websites of all 53 Member States. The grey literature searches of websites encompassed 14 European languages (Bosnian, Catalan, Croatian, Dutch, English, French, German, Italian, Montenegrin, Romanian, Russian, Serbian, Slovene and Spanish), which would encompass many Member

States; however, the review might still have missed some specific literature from eastern European/central Asian countries.

### 3.1.3 Quality of the data and contradictory information

The reported availability of nutritional and health information labels in the WHO European Region and the data given in Annex 2 (Tables A2.1 and A2.2) are based on data reported by Member States in the WHO survey (76), information from the literature review and the data reported by the alcohol industry on their voluntary commitments. However, there have been cases where EU countries have reported the presence of labelling in a survey to the EU but not in a survey for WHO, or vice versa, and where no other information could be found. Similarly, the lack of reports for alcohol industry commitments with clearly detailed methodology on the implementation of the pledges might raise doubts on actual implementation. It is difficult, therefore, to have a complete picture of the true presence of labelling in the Region.

In addition to the lack of unified and reliable data sources for the WHO European Region, laws related to alcohol labelling (particularly nutritional information) may also be embedded in non-alcohol control laws (such as food packaging). The situation varies from country to country, making it harder to uncover the relevant information during searching. This might have led to some gaps in the resulting picture of nutritional labelling for alcoholic beverages in the Region, particularly if no other documents referring to this were available.

## 3.2 Ensuring the rights to consumer information through labelling

The review clearly highlights that a large proportion of consumers in the WHO European Region do not have access to ingredients and health information in labels on alcoholic beverages, contrary to the case for other similar products. While some health messages are available, these tend to target only specific groups and might be misunderstood by consumers to mean that alcohol is only a risk for those in a specific group, such as pregnant women or underage drinkers. Given the rights of consumers, and as done with other carcinogenic products harmful for all the population, messages should clearly reflect the risks of alcohol consumption to all and provide warnings to all consumers about its harms (e.g. as for tobacco). Moreover, given the right to consumer information in Europe, the scaling up of mandatory labelling seems a worrying omission in most countries. Examples of success in this review highlight government-led regulation as an effective route by which countries can ensure that WHO recommendations are followed, and labelling of alcoholic beverages becomes a reality.

## 3.3 Ensuring adequate and independent monitoring

The review shows a strong need for a more thorough system of information provision, monitoring, evaluation and mechanisms to enforce implementation.

**Information collection and monitoring.** There is a need for an improved system of information collection regarding mandatory labelling and its implementation in the Member States of the WHO European Region that goes beyond indicating the presence or absence of an indicator for the WHO Global Information System on Alcohol and Health (76) or the country status reports. Monitoring the relevant regulations and reporting on implementation progress should not be left solely to industry or civil society organizations. The same applies for voluntary commitments, where an independent system for reporting, with a set of commonly agreed indicators and methodology, should be set.

**Independent auditing.** An independent system for auditing what is actually present on the labels, similar to that identified in two papers for this report (71,129), should be developed and undertaken across countries in the WHO European Region to monitor to what extent the provisions in regulations or voluntary commitments are implemented. A centrally developed framework and toolkit for helping with monitoring and enforcement might be a first step in establishing a homogeneous common ground. This is particularly important for industry-led labelling, where currently there is no independent reporting and monitoring of implementation. Such effective auditing becomes particularly relevant given the myriad of different commitments and claims of alcohol labelling at national and supranational levels and the lack of independent evidence on industry-led action. Such monitoring systems would also serve as indirect incentives for enforcement of implementation, particularly if the systems were linked to penetration of the messages.

**Evaluation.** Evaluation of the impact of labelling policies and actions is missing overall in the WHO European Region, and strong efforts are needed, as for tobacco, to ensure the use of the most effective messages and improvement of the less effective ones so that labelling is as impactful across populations as it can be. Evaluation of what helps with enforcement of labelling implementation would also provide the necessary background to help to accelerate efforts and get it right, as experienced for tobacco.

**Access to lessons learned.** Finally, there is a need to further understand the processes of developing labelling regulations and ensuring their implementation, using lessons learned by different stakeholders, in order to inform further attempts in policy-making. This report is a first step in that direction.

## 3.4 Policy considerations

Based on the findings of this review, the main policy and practice considerations in the WHO European Region for the development of nutritional and health information labelling on alcohol products are to:

- establish labelling that includes all recommended nutritional values and lists all ingredients;
- establish labelling that includes the harm done by alcohol relevant to the whole population (e.g. cancer), pregnancy-related harm, harm to minors, drinking and driving warnings, and recommendations on lower-risk drinking guidelines indicated as standard drinks in countries where this would be applicable;
- ensure regulations include specific directions about how all information should be presented on labels (e.g. appropriate size and font, front of pack, rotating messages and easy-to-understand information), ideally following WHO recommendations;
- favour mandatory regulation over voluntary commitments as this allows better control over the content and presentation of the message, presentation of stronger evidence and more assurance of good penetration of labelling;
- provide clear input and direction from public health bodies if messages are to be voluntary and self-regulated by industry to ensure that effective messages are displayed;
- consider introducing any specific labelling policy as a part of an existing or new larger policy package and using a stepwise approach to facilitate achieving a full labelling policy;
- leverage facilitating contextual factors when developing policy (e.g. public support, political will and/or evidence of alcohol-related harm in the country) and use the best policy window to put proposals forward for the introduction of labelling;

- expect some barriers to the development of legislation, such as opposition from the alcohol industry or delays in processes of international bodies, and have strong counterarguments prepared in advance to best support the proposed legislation;
- ensure that mechanisms for enforcing implementation, for independent monitoring and for evaluation of the impact of labelling policies are in place regardless of whether labelling is voluntary or mandatory; and
- invest in strengthening research on alcohol labelling to identify the most effective form and content of the labelling communication (e.g. photographs, pictograms and written messages, including the most effective wording).

## 4. CONCLUSIONS

The WHO European Region has the highest levels of per capita alcohol consumption, with 10% of all deaths attributable to alcohol. Given alcohol-associated harms, providing consumer information about its risks through product labelling, a WHO recommendation, is paramount. Labelling is already mandatory for consumer products such as non-alcoholic beverages, foodstuffs and tobacco.

Of the Member States of the Region, only 40% have some legislation on ingredients listing, 19% have some legislation on nutritional values and 28% have some legislation on some aspects of health information labelling, focusing mainly on pregnancy and underage drinking. Voluntary industry commitments, although increasing in amount and scope, either are not monitored transparently or do not meet the recommendations in the WHO discussion paper on policy options for alcohol labelling.

The existence of legislation or an industry commitment does not ensure implementation is enforced, has the expected reach or follows recommendations for the presentation of messages on the labels. Independent monitoring and evaluation of existing/new measures are essential to understand the impact, improve recommendations and strengthen future labelling decisions.

Research suggests that national policies, influenced by the alcohol industry, are not consistent nor absolute when it comes to alcohol warning labels and do not account for public health interests. For the tobacco industry, warning labels are mandated for tobacco products despite continued challenges by the industry; these products cause 7 million deaths every year yet similar warnings are not mandated for alcohol products, which cause 3 million deaths a year. This begs the question: how many more deaths does it take to justify a label?

# REFERENCES

1. GBD 2016 Risk Factors Collaborators. Global, regional, and national comparative risk assessment of 84 behavioural, environmental and occupational, and metabolic risks or clusters of risks, 1990–2016: a systematic analysis for the Global Burden of Disease Study 2016. Lancet. 2017;390(10100):1345–422. doi: 10.1016/S0140-6736(17)32366-8.

2. Global status report on alcohol and health 2018. Geneva: World Health Organization; 2018 (https://apps.who.int/iris/bitstream/handle/10665/274603/9789241565639-eng.pdf?ua=1, accessed 11 December 2019).

3. Alcohol status report 2018: alcohol consumption, harm and policy responses in 30 countries. Copenhagen: WHO Regional Office for Europe; 2018 (http://www.euro.who.int/__data/assets/pdf_file/0019/411418/Alcohol-consumption-harm-policy-responses-30-European-countries-2019.pdf?ua=1, accessed 16 December 2019).

4. Alcohol consumption and ethyl carbamate. In: IARC monographs on the evaluation of carcinogenic risks to humans, vol 96. Lyon: International Agency for Research on Cancer; 2010.

5. LoConte NK, Brewster AM, Kaur JS, Merrill JK, Alberg AJ. Alcohol and cancer: a statement of the American Society of Clinical Oncology. J Clin Oncol. 2018;36(1):83–93. doi: 10.1200/JCO.2017.76.1155.

6. Rehm J, Gmel Sr GE, Gmel G, Hasan OSM, Imtiaz S, Popova S et al. The relationship between different dimensions of alcohol use and the burden of disease: an update. Addiction. 2017;112(6):968–1001. doi: 10.1111/add.13757.

7. Millwood IY, Walters RG, Mei XW, Guo Y, Yang L, Bian Z et al. Conventional and genetic evidence on alcohol and vascular disease aetiology: a prospective study of 500 000 men and women in China. Lancet. 2019;393(10183):1831–42. doi: 10.1016/S0140-6736(18)31772-0.

8. Imtiaz S, Shield KD, Roerecke M, Samokhvalov AV, Lönnroth K, Rehm J. Alcohol consumption as a risk factor for tuberculosis: meta-analyses and burden of disease. Eur Respir J. 2017;50(1):pii:1700216. doi: 10.1183/13993003.00216-2017.

9. Rehm J, Probst C, Shield KD, Shuper PA. Does alcohol use have a causal effect on HIV incidence and disease progression? A review of the literature and a modeling strategy for quantifying the effect. Popul Health Metr. 2017;15(1):4. doi: 10.1186/s12963-017-0121-9.

10. Boden JM, Fergusson DM. Alcohol and depression. Addiction. 2011;106(5):906–14. doi: 10.1111/j.1360-0443.2010.03351.x.

11. Hasin DS, Grant BF. Major depression in 6050 former drinkers: association with past alcohol dependence. Arch Gen Psychiatry. 2002;59(9):794–800. doi: 10.1001/archpsyc.59.9.794.

12. Wood AM, Kaptoge S, Butterworth AS, Willeit P, Warnakula S, Bolton T et al. Risk thresholds for alcohol consumption: combined analysis of individual-participant data for 599 912 current drinkers in 83 prospective studies. Lancet. 2018;391(10129):1513–23. doi: 10.1016/S0140-6736(18)30134-X.

13. Griswold MG, Fullman N, Hawley C, Arian N, Zimsen SRM, Tymeson HD et al. Alcohol use and burden for 195 countries and territories, 1990–2016: a systematic analysis for the Global Burden of Disease Study 2016. Lancet. 2018;392(10152):1015–35. doi: 10.1016/S0140-6736(18)31310-2.

14. Donnelly PD, Ward CL. Interpersonal violence and its importance as a global public health issue. In: Donnelly PD, Ward CL, editors. Oxford textbook of violence prevention: epidemiology, evidence, and policy. Oxford: Oxford University Press; 2015:3–8.

15. Brown W, Leonard KE. Does alcohol cause violence and aggression? In: Sturmey P, editor. The Wiley handbook of violence and aggression. Hoboken (NJ): Wiley-Blackwell; 2017:1-13.

16. Anderson P, Baumberg B. Alcohol in Europe. London: Institute of Alcohol Studies; 2006 (https://ec.europa.eu/health/archive/ph_determinants/life_style/alcohol/documents/alcohol_europe_en.pdf, accessed 11 December 2019).

17. Canadian Substance Use Costs and Harms Scientific Working Group. Canadian substance use costs and harms (2007–2014). Ottawa: Canadian Centre on Substance Use and Addiction; 2018 (https://www.ccsa.ca/sites/default/files/2019-04/CSUCH-Canadian-Substance-Use-Costs-Harms-Report-2018-en.pdf, accessed 11 December 2019).

18. Petticrew M, Shemilt I, Lorenc T, Marteau TM, Melendez-Torres GJ, O'Mara-Eves A et al. Alcohol advertising and public health: systems perspectives versus narrow perspectives. J Epidemiol Community Health. 2017;71(3):308–12. doi: 10.1136/jech-2016-207644.

19. European action plan to reduce the harmful use of alcohol 2012–2020. Copenhagen: WHO Regional Office for Europe; 2011 (http://www.euro.who.int/__data/assets/pdf_file/0008/178163/E96726.pdf, accessed 11 December 2019).

20. Global strategy to reduce the harmful use of alcohol. Geneva: World Health Organization; 2010 (https://www.who.int/substance_abuse/msbalcstragegy.pdf, accessed 11 December 2019).

21. O'Brien P, Mitchell AD. On the bottle: health information, alcohol labelling and the WTO technical barriers to trade agreement. QUT Law Rev. 2018;18:124–5. doi: 10.5204/qutlr.v18i1.732.

22. Cecchini M, Warin L. Impact of food labelling systems on food choices and eating behaviours: a systematic review and meta-analysis of randomized studies. Obes Rev. 2016;17(3):201–10. doi: 10.1111/obr.12364.

23. Shangguan S, Afshin A, Shulkin M, Ma W, Marsden D, Smith J et al. A meta-analysis of food labeling effects on consumer diet behaviors and industry practices. Am J Prev Med. 2019;56(2):300–14. doi: 10.1016/j.amepre.2018.09.024.

24. Hammond D. Health warning messages on tobacco products: a review. Tob Control. 2011;20(5):327–37. doi: 10.1136/tc.2010.037630.

25. Noar SM, Francis DB, Bridges C, Sontag JM, Ribisl KM, Brewer NT. The impact of strengthening cigarette pack warnings: systematic review of longitudinal observational studies. Soc Sci Med. 2016;164:118–29. doi: 10.1016/j.socscimed.2016.06.011.

26. Wilkinson C, Room R. Warnings on alcohol containers and advertisements: international experience and evidence on effects. Drug Alcohol Rev. 2009;28(4):426–35. doi: 10.1111/j.1465-3362.2009.00055.x.

27. Wilkinson C, Allsop S, Cail D, Chikritzhs T, Daube M, Kirby G et al. Alcohol warning labels: evidence of effectiveness on risky alcohol consumption and short term outcomes. Curtin: National Drug Research Institute; 2009 (https://www.foodstandards.gov.au/code/applications/documents/Alcohol-warning-labels-report-1.pdf, accessed 11 December 2019).

28. Scholes-Balog KE, Heerde JA, Hemphill SA. Alcohol warning labels: unlikely to affect alcohol-related beliefs and behaviours in adolescents. Aust N Z J Public Health. 2012;36(6):524–9. doi: 10.1111/j.1753-6405.2012.00934.x.

29. Hassan L, Shiu E. A systematic review of the efficacy of alcohol warning labels: insights from qualitative and quantitative research in the new millennium. J Soc Mark. 2018;8(3):333–52. doi: 10.1108/JSOCM-03-2017-0020.

30. Purmehdi M, Legoux R, Carrillat F, Senecal S. The effectiveness of warning labels for consumers: a meta-analytic investigation into their

underlying process and contingencies. J Public Policy Mark. 2017;36(1):36–53. doi: 10.1509/jppm.14.047.

31. Osiowy M, Stockwell T, Zhao J, Thompson K, Moore S. How much did you actually drink last night? An evaluation of standard drink labels as an aid to monitoring personal consumption. Addict Res Theory. 2015;23(2):163–9. doi: 10.3109/16066359.2014.955480.

32. Wettlaufer A. Can a label help me drink in moderation? A review of the evidence on standard drink labelling. Subst Use Misuse. 2018;53(4):585–95. doi: 10.1080/10826084.2017.1349798.

33. Hobin E, Vallance K, Zuo F, Stockwell T, Rosella L, Simniceanu A et al. Testing the efficacy of alcohol labels with standard drink information and national drinking guidelines on consumers' ability to estimate alcohol consumption. Alcohol Alcohol. 2018;53(1):3–11. doi: 10.1093/alcalc/agx052.

34. Vallance K, Romanovska I, Stockwell T, Hammond D, Rosella L, Hobin E. "We have a right to know": exploring consumer opinions on content, design and acceptability of enhanced alcohol labels. Alcohol Alcohol. 2018;53(1):20–5. doi: 10.1093/alcalc/agx068.

35. Stockwell T. A review of research into the impacts of alcohol warning labels on attitudes and behaviour. Victoria: Centre for Addictions Research of BC; 2006 (https://www.uvic.ca/research/centres/cisur/assets/docs/report-impacts-alcohol-warning-labels.pdf, accessed 11 December 2019).

36. Kelly B, Jewell J. What is the evidence on the policy specifications, development processes and effectiveness of existing front-of-pack food labelling policies in the WHO European Region? Copenhagen: WHO Regional Office for Europe; 2018 (Health Evidence Network (HEN) synthesis report 61; http://www.euro.who.int/__data/assets/pdf_file/0007/384460/Web-WHO-HEN-Report-61-on-FOPL.pdf?ua=1, accessed 11 December 2019).

37. Thomas G, Gonneau G, Poole N, Cook J. The effectiveness of alcohol warning labels in the prevention of fetal alcohol spectrum disorder: a brief review. Int J Alcohol Drug Res. 2014;3(1):91–103. doi: 10.7895/ijadr.v3i1.126.

38. Louise J, Eliott J, Olver I, Braunack-Mayer A. Mandatory cancer risk warnings on alcoholic beverages: what are the ethical issues? Am J Bioeth. 2015;15(3):3–11. doi: 10.1080/15265161.2014.998373.

39. Hassan L, Shiu E. Communicating messages about drinking. Alcohol Alcohol. 2018;53(1):1–2. doi: 10.1093/alcalc/agx112.

40. Joint FAO/WHO Food Standards Programme Codex Committee on Food Labelling, 45th session, Ottawa, 13–17 May 2019. Rome: Joint Food and Agriculture Organization of the United Nations/World Health Organization Food Standards Programme; 2019 (http://www.fao.org/fao-who-codexalimentarius/sh-proxy/en/?lnk=1&url=https%253A%252F%252Fworkspace.fao.org%252Fsites%252Fcodex%252FMeetings%252FCX-714-45%252Ffl45_01e.pdf, accessed 11 December 2019).

41. Codex Alimentarius. Guidelines on nutrition labelling CAC/GL 2-1985. Rome: Joint Food and Agriculture Organization of the United Nations/World Health Organization Food Standards Programme; 2017 (http://www.fao.org/fao-who-codexalimentarius/sh-proxy/en/?lnk=1&url=https%253A%252F%252Fworkspace.fao.org%252Fsites%252Fcodex%252FStandards%252FCXG%2B2-1985%252FCXG_002e.pdf, accessed 11 December 2019).

42. Codex Alimentarius Commission. General standard for the labelling of prepackaged foods. Rome: Joint Food and Agriculture Organization of the United Nations/World Health Organization Food Standards Programme; 2018 (http://www.fao.org/fao-who-codexalimentarius/sh-proxy/en/?lnk=1&url=https%253A%252F%252Fworkspace.fao.org%252Fsites%252Fcodex%252FStandards%252FCXS%2B1-1985%252FCXS_001e.pdf, accessed 11 December 2019).

43. González-Vaqué L. Self-regulation of the labelling of the list of ingredients of alcoholic beverages: a long-term solution? Eur Food Feed Law Rev. 2017;12(5):413–21.

44. Martin-Moreno JM, Harris ME, Breda J, Moller L, Alfonso-Sanchez JL, Gorgojo L. Enhanced labelling on alcoholic drinks: reviewing the evidence to guide alcohol policy. Eur J Public Health. 2013;23(6):1082–7. doi: 10.1093/eurpub/ckt046.

45. Mitchell MC, Herlong HF. Alcohol and nutrition: caloric value, bioenergetics, and relationship to liver damage. Annu Rev Nutr. 1986;6(1):457–74. doi: 10.1146/annurev.nu.06.070186.002325.

46. Tolstrup JS, Heitmann BL, Tjønneland AM, Overvad OK, Sørensen TIA, Grønbaek MN. The relation between drinking pattern and body mass index and waist and hip circumference. Int J Obes. 2005;29(5):490–7. doi: 10.1038/sj.ijo.0802874.

47. Schröder H, Morales-Molina JA, Bermejo S, Barral D, Mándoli ES, Grau M et al. Relationship of abdominal obesity with alcohol consumption at population scale. Eur J Nutr. 2007;46(7):369–76. doi: 10.1007/s00394-007-0674-7.

48. Wannamethee SG, Shaper AG, Whincup PH. Alcohol and adiposity: effects of quantity and type of drink and time relation with meals. Int J Obes. 2005;29(12):1436–44. doi: 10.1038/sj.ijo.0803034.

49. Arif AA, Rohrer JE. Patterns of alcohol drinking and its association with obesity: data from the Third National Health and Nutrition Examination Survey, 1988–1994. BMC Public Health. 2005;5(1):126. doi: 10.1186/1471-2458-5-126.

50. Lukasiewicz E, Mennen LI, Bertrais S, Arnault N, Preziosi P, Galan P et al. Alcohol intake in relation to body mass index and waist-to-hip ratio: the importance of type of alcoholic beverage. Public Health Nutr. 2005;8(3):315–20. doi: 10.1079/phn2004680.

51. Wang L, Lee I-M, Manson JE, Buring JE, Sesso HD. Alcohol consumption, weight gain, and risk of becoming overweight in middle-aged and older women. Arch Intern Med. 2010;170(5):453–61. doi: 10.1001/archinternmed.2009.527.

52. Nielsen SJ, Kit BK, Fakhouri T, Ogden CL. Calories consumed from alcoholic beverages by US adults, 2007–2010. NCHS Data Brief. 2012 Nov;(110):1–8.

53. Yeomans MR. Alcohol, appetite and energy balance: is alcohol intake a risk factor for obesity? Physiol Behav. 2010;100(1):82–9. doi: 10.1016/j.physbeh.2010.01.012.

54. Shelton NJ, Knott CS. Association between alcohol calorie intake and overweight and obesity in English adults. Am J Public Health. 2014;104(4):629–31. doi: 10.2105/AJPH.2013.301643.

55. Traversy G, Chaput JP. Alcohol consumption and obesity: an update. Curr Obes Rep. 2015;4(1):122–30. doi: 10.1007/s13679-014-0129-4.

56. Hart CL, Morrison DS, Batty GD, Mitchell RJ, Smith GD. Effect of body mass index and alcohol consumption on liver disease: analysis of data from two prospective cohort studies. BMJ. 2010;340:c1240. doi: 10.1136/bmj.c1240.

57. Buykx P, Gilligan C, Ward B, Kippen R, Chapman K. Public support for alcohol policies associated with knowledge of cancer risk. Int J Drug Policy. 2015;26(4):371–9. doi: 10.1016/j.drugpo.2014.08.006.

58. Scheideler JK, Klein WMP. Awareness of the link between alcohol consumption and cancer across the world: a review. Cancer Epidemiol Biomarkers Prev. 2018;27(4):429–37. doi: 10.1158/1055-9965.EPI-17-0645.

59. Al-Hamdani M. The case for stringent alcohol warning labels: lessons from the tobacco control experience. J Public Health Policy. 2014;35(1):65–74. doi: 10.1057/jphp.2013.47.

60. Pettigrew S, Jongenelis M, Chikritzhs T, Slevin T, Pratt IS, Glance D et al. Developing cancer warning statements for alcoholic beverages. BMC Public Health. 2014;14(1):786. doi: 10.1186/1471-2458-14-786.

61. Zahra D, Monk RL, Corder E. "IF you drink alcohol, THEN you will get cancer": investigating how reasoning accuracy is affected by pictorially presented graphic alcohol warnings. Alcohol Alcohol. 2015;50(5):608–16. doi: 10.1093/alcalc/agv029.

62. Alcohol labelling: a discussion document on policy options. Copenhagen: WHO Regional Office for Europe; 2017 (http://www.euro.who.int/en/health-topics/disease-prevention/alcohol-use/publications/2017/alcohol-labelling-a-discussion-document-on-policy-options-2017, accessed 11 December 2019).

63. Regulation (EU) No 1169/2011 of the European Parliament and of the Council of 25 October 2011 on the provision of food information to consumers. OJ. 2011;L 304/18 (https://eur-lex.europa.eu/legal-content/EN/TXT/PDF/?uri=CELEX:32011R1169&from=EN, accessed 6 January 2020).

64. Consumer labelling and alcoholic drinks. Hamm: Deutsche Hauptstelle für Suchtfragen eV; 2008 (https://www.dhs.de/fileadmin/user_upload/pdf/Pathways_for_Health-Project/consumer_labelling_report.pdf, accessed 11 December 2019).

65. A brief summary of health warning labels on alcoholic beverages. Brussels: Eurocare; 2009 (https://www.eurocare.org/media/GENERAL/docs/reports/overviewlabellinginitiativeseurocare2009.pdf, accessed 11 December 2019).

66. What's not on the bottle? Eurocare reflections on alcohol labelling. Brussels: Eurocare; 2014 (https://www.eurocare.org/media/GENERAL/docs/reports/2014novwhatsnotonthebottleeurocarereflectionsonalcohollabelling.pdf, accessed 11 December 2019).

67. Farke W. Health warnings and responsibility messages on alcoholic beverages: a review of practices in Europe. Brussels: Eurocare; 2011.

68. Report from the Commission to the European Parliament and the Council regarding the mandatory labelling of the list of ingredients and the nutrition declaration of alcoholic beverages. Brussels: European Commission; 2017 (https://ec.europa.eu/food/sites/food/files/safety/docs/fs_labelling-nutrition_legis_alcohol-report_en.pdf, accessed 11 December 2019).

69. Taylor L. Alcohol warning labels in the UK. J Food Prod Mark. 2006;21(1):103–14. doi: 10.1300/J038v12n01_07.

70. Mayor S. Ministers may legislate after finding 85% of labels on alcohol to be inadequate. BMJ. 2010;340:c966. doi: 10.1136/bmj.c966.

71. Petticrew M, Douglas N, Knai C, Durand MA, Eastmure E, Mays N. Health information on alcoholic beverage containers: has the alcohol industry's pledge in England to improve labelling been met? Addiction. 2016;111(1):51–5. doi: 10.1111/add.13094.

72. Petticrew M, Douglas N, Knai C, Hessari NM, Durand MA, Eastmure E et al. Provision of information to consumers about the calorie content of alcoholic drinks: did the Responsibility Deal pledge by alcohol retailers and producers increase the availability of calorie information? Public Health. 2017;149:159–66. doi: 10.1016/j.puhe.2017.04.020.

73. Dumas A, Toutain S, Simmat-Durand L. The French paradox: forbidding alcohol during pregnancy, but making an exception for wine! In: Hoffman JD, editor. Pregnancy and alcohol consumption. Hauppage (NY): Nova Science; 2010:245–61.

74. Dossou G, Gallopel-Morvan K, Diouf J-F. The effectiveness of current French health warnings displayed on alcohol advertisements and alcoholic beverages. Eur J Public Health. 2017;27(4):699–704. doi: 10.1093/eurpub/ckw263.

75. Gornall J. Alcohol and public health. Europe under the influence. BMJ. 2014;348:g1166. doi: 10.1136/bmj.g1166.

76. Warning and consumer information labels. In: Information system on alcohol and health (GISAH) [website]. Geneva: World Health Organization; 2018 (http://apps.who.int/gho/data/node.gisah.A1191?lang=en&showonly=GISAH, accessed 11 December 2019).

77. Beverage alcohol labelling requirements [website]. London: International Alliance for Responsible Drinking; 2019 (http://www.iard.org/resources/beverage-alcohol-labeling-requirements/, accessed 11 December 2019).

78. EU-food information regulation 1169/2011: implementing measures by Member States. Brussels: Food Lawyers' Network Worldwide; 2015.

79. Scotch Whisky Association: written evidence. In: House of Commons Treasury Committee inquiry: the economic and financial costs and benefits of the UK's EU membership. London: House of Commons Treasury Committee;

2016:43 (https://publications.parliament.uk/pa/cm201617/cmselect/cmtreasy/122/122.pdf, accessed 11 December 2019).

80. [Technical regulations EAEU TR 047/2018 on the safety of alcoholic beverages]. Moscow: Eurasian Customs Union; 2018 (in Russian; https://docs.eaeunion.org/docs/ru-ru/01420230/cncd_10122018_98, accessed 11 December 2019).

81. LOI No. 2005-102 du 11 février 2005 pour l'égalité des droits et des chances, la participation et la citoyenneté des personnes handicapées (1). Paris: Légifrance; 2005 (https://www.legifrance.gouv.fr/affichTexte.do?cidTexte=JORFTEXT000000809647&categorieLien=id, accessed 6 January 2020).

82. Jugendschutzgesetz. Berlin: Bundesministeriums der Justiz und für Verbraucherschutz; 2002 (https://www.gesetze-im-internet.de/juschg/BJNR273000002.html, accessed 6 January 2020).

83. Public Health (Alcohol) Act 2018. Dublin: Government of Ireland; 2018 (https://data.oireachtas.ie/ie/oireachtas/act/2018/24/eng/enacted/a2418.pdf, accessed 11 December 2019).

84. Warning on alcohol bottles and in advertisements for alcohol. Jerusalem: State of Israel Ministry of Health; 30 July 2013 (press release; https://www.health.gov.il/English/News_and_Events/Spokespersons_Messages/Pages/30072013_1.aspx, accessed 6 January 2020).

85. [Order No. 4-527 on the approval of the rules on the labelling of alcoholic beverages with principles of alcoholic behaviour for pregnant women]. Vilnius: Government of the Republic of Lithuania; 2016 (in Lithuanian; https://e-seimas.lrs.lt/portal/legalAct/lt/TAD/853d0b006a3511e6a421ea2bde782b94?positionInSearchResults=0&searchModelUUID=c99381d3-c520-43c4-8653-0807a80d5dbe, accessed 6 January 2020).

86. Representantforslag om en offensiv og solidarisk alkoholpolitikk [Representative proposal on an offensive and solidarity alcohol policy]. Oslo: Stortinget; 2019 (Dokument 8:141 S (2017–2018, Innst. 38 S (2018–2019), in Norwegian; https://www.stortinget.no/no/Saker-og-publikasjoner/Saker/Sak/?p=71296, accessed 6 January 2020).

87. Lege Nr. 1100 cu privire la fabricarea şi circulaţia alcoolului etilic şi a producţiei alcoolice [Law No. 1100 on the manufacture and circulation of ethyl alcohol and alcoholic beverages]. Chişinău: Republic of Moldova; 2000 (in Romanian; http://lex.justice.md/viewdoc.php?action=view&view=doc&id=334893&lang=1, accessed 6 January 2020).

88. Communiqué on warning messages to be affixed on the packaging of alcoholic beverages. Ankara: Republic of Turkey; 2013 (https://members.wto.org/crnattachments/2013/tbt/TUR/13_3072_00_e.pdf, accessed 6 January 2020).

89. [Technical regulation on food products labelling]. Moscow: Eurasian Customs Union; 2011 (TR SU 022/2011, in Russian; http://www.eurasiancommission.org/ru/act/texnreg/deptexreg/tr/Documents/TrTsPishevkaMarkirovka.pdf, accessed 11 December 2019).

90. [Technical regulation on food safety]. Moscow: Eurasian Customs Union; 2018 (TR SU 021/2011, in Russian; http://www.eurasiancommission.org/ru/act/texnreg/deptexreg/tr/Documents/TR TS PishevayaProd.pdf, accessed 6 January 2020).

91. On the adoption of the technical regulations TR CU 021/2011 of the Customs Union on food safety (as amended on 10 June 2014)]. Moscow: Customs Union Commission; 2018 (http://www.eurexcert.com/TRCUpdf/TRCU-0021-On-food-safety.pdf, accessed 28 January 2020).

92. [Alcohol labelling requirements changed]. Nur-Sultan: Atameken [National Chamber of Entrepreneurs of the Republic of Kazakhstan]; 28 October 2014 (in Russian; https://atameken.kz/ru/news/11778-11778, accessed 11 December 2019).

93. [Technical regulation on safety of alcoholic beverages]. Moscow: Eurasian Customs Union; 2018 (in Russian; http://www.eurasiancommission.org/ru/act/texnreg/deptexreg/tr/Documents/ТР ТС Алкоголь ВГС.pdf, accessed 11 December 2019).

94. Minutes of the meeting of 18–19 March 2015. Geneva: World Trade Organization Committee on Technical Barriers to Trade; 2015 (https://docs.wto.org/dol2fe/Pages/FE_Search/FE_S_S009-DP.aspx?language=E&CatalogueIdList=134466,132661,132294, 130728,130294&CurrentCatalogueIdIndex=2&FullTextHash=&HasEnglishRecord=True&HasFrenchRecord= True&HasSpanishRecord=True, accessed 11 December 2019).

95. Anheuser-Busch InBev. Informing consumers about beer ingredients and nutritional values. Brussels: European Alcohol and Health Forum; 2015 (https://webgate.ec.europa.eu/sanco/heidi/eahf/commitment/view/1720, accessed 11 December 2019).

96. Heineken. Provision of nutritional and ingredients information to consumers on label for all Heineken beers in Europe. Brussels: Commitment to European

Alcohol and Health Forum; 2015 (https://webgate.ec.europa.eu/sanco/heidi/eahf/commitment/view/1722, accessed 11 December 2019).

97. Diageo consumer information standards. London: Diageo; 2016 (https://www.diageo.com/en/investors/financial-results-and-presentations/diageo-consumer-information-standards-summary/, accessed 11 December 2019).

98. Johnnie Walker to provide per serving alcohol content and nutritional information on-pack. London: Diageo; 2016 (https://www.diageo.com/en/news-and-media/press-releases/johnnie-walker-to-provide-per-serving-alcohol-content-and-nutritional-information-on-pack/, accessed 11 December 2019).

99. Guinness becomes first global beverage brand to provide consumers with on-label alcohol and nutritional content. London: Diageo; 2017 (https://www.diageo.com/PR1346/aws/media/3807/guinness-labelling-press-release.pdf, accessed 11 December 2019).

100. Third report: 2012–2015. European beer pledge: a package of responsibility initiatives from Europe's brewers. Brussels: The Brewers of Europe; 2017 (https://brewersofeurope.org/uploads/mycms-files/documents/publications/2017/beer_pledge_web.pdf, accessed 11 December 2019).

101. Beer calories to be printed on labels. Helsinki: The Federation of the Brewing and Soft Drinks Industry; 2008 (http://www.panimoliitto.fi/en/beer-calories-to-be-printed-on-labels/, accessed 11 December 2019).

102. Mærkning på øl [Labelling on beer]. Copenhagen: Danish Brewers' Association; 2012 (in Danish; https://www.bryggeriforeningen.dk/ol/fodevarer/maerkning/, accessed 11 December 2019).

103. Genstandsmærkning [Object labelling]. Copenhagen: Danish Brewers' Association; 2012 (in Danish; https://www.bryggeriforeningen.dk/ol/sundhed/genstandsmaerkning/, accessed 11 December 2019).

104. Etiketteringshandleiding bij Verordening 1169/2011 [Labelling manual regulation 1169/2011]. Schenkkade: Nederlandse Brouwers; 2018 (in Dutch; https://www.nederlandsebrouwers.nl/site/assets/files/1382/handleiding_nederlandse_brouwers_bij_etiketteringsverordening_1169-2011_februari_2018.pdf, accessed 11 December 2019).

105. European Cider and Fruit Wine Association. Voluntary ingredient listing and nutrition information: production process for cider and fruit wine.

    Brussels: European Commission; 2018 (https://ec.europa.eu/food/sites/food/files/safety/docs/fs_labelling-nutrition_legis_alcohol-self-regulatory-proposal_cider_en.pdf, accessed 11 December 2019).

106. What's in a beer? European brewers' commitment to listing ingredients and nutrition information. Brussels: The Brewers of Europe; 2015 (https://beerwisdom.eu/wp-content/uploads/2018/03/whats-in-beer-20180312-1.pdf, accessed 11 December 2019).

107. Detailed wine and aromatised wine products annex to the self-regulatory proposal from the European alcoholic beverages sectors on the provision of nutrition information and ingredients. Brussels: European Commission; 2018 (https://ec.europa.eu/food/sites/food/files/safety/docs/fs_labelling-nutrition_legis_alcohol-self-regulatory-proposal_annex-wine-en.pdf, accessed 11 December 2019).

108. Self-regulatory proposal from the European alcoholic beverages sectors on the provision of nutrition information and ingredients listing. Brussels: European Commission; 2017 (https://ec.europa.eu/food/sites/food/files/safety/docs/fs_labelling-nutrition_legis_alcohol-self-regulatory-proposal_en.pdf, accessed 11 December 2019).

109. Spirits sector annex to the self-regulatory proposal from the European alcoholic beverages sectors on the provision of nutrition information and ingredients listing. Brussels: spiritsEUROPE; 2018 (https://ec.europa.eu/food/sites/food/files/safety/docs/fs_labelling-nutrition_legis_alcohol-self-regulatory-proposal_annex-spirits-en.pdf, accessed 6 January 2020).

110. All beers should be labelling ingredients and calories by end 2022. Brussels: The Brewers of Europe; 13 June 2019 (https://brewersofeurope.org/site/media-centre/post.php?doc_id=975, accessed 11 December 2019).

111. Consumer information: European producers sign memorandum of understanding to provide energy value on spirit drinks. Brussels: spiritsEUROPE; 4 June 2019 (https://spirits.eu/media/press-releases/consumer-information-european-producers-sign-memorandum-of-understanding-to-provide-energy-value-on-spirit-drinks, accessed 11 December 2019).

112. Beer, wine and spirits producers' commitments: combating harmful drinking. 2017 progress report and five-year summary of actions. London: International Alliance for Responsible Drinking; 2018 (https://www.iard.org/getattachment/61806635-0fc1-4dbb-a816-92dd167de8d1/2017-producers-commitments-full-report.pdf, accessed 11 December 2019).

113. The placement of the French pregnancy logo on the back label of all of Pernod Ricard's wine and spirit brands in the EU-27 countries. In: Annual Report 2007/2008. Paris: Pernod Ricard SA; 2008:93 (https://www.pernod-ricard.com/en/download/file/fid/8051/, accessed 11 December 2019).

114. Anheuser-Busch InBev. Pictorial labelling commitment (submission 1323905857765-1484). Brussels: European Alcohol and Health Forum; 2011 (https://webcache.googleusercontent.com/search?q=cache:Oi5OO_0w2sUJ:https://webgate.ec.europa.eu/sanco/heidi/eahf/commitment/view/1484+&cd=1&hl=en&ct=clnk&gl=nl, accessed 6 January 2020).

115. Marketing communication policy. Copenhagen: Carlsberg Breweries; 2017 (https://carlsberggroup.com/media/17989/marketing-communication-policy.pdf, accessed 11 December 2019).

116. Tufts global alcohol labelling guidance project. Boston (MA): Tufts School of Medicine; 2018 (https://globalguidancelabel.publichealth.tufts.edu/, accessed 11 December 2019).

117. Labelling, informing, marketing: commitment report. Woking: SAB Miller; 2014 (https://www.ab-inbev.com/content/dam/universaltemplate/ab-inbev/investors/sabmiller/reports/other-reports/labelling-informing-marketing-commitment-report-2014.pdf, accessed 11 December 2019).

118. Regulations on alcohol marketing. Portugal: European Centre for Monitoring Alcohol Marketing; 2018 (https://eucam.info/regulations-on-alcohol-marketing/, accessed 11 December 2019).

119. [About the Responsibility Alliance]. Greece: The Alcoholic Drinks Association Responsibility Alliance; 2018 (in Greek; http://responsibility-alliance.gr/#members%0A, accessed 11 December 2019).

120. Sweden to introduce booze warning labels. The Local. 9 July 2007 (http://www.thelocal.se/7833/20070709/, accessed 11 December 2019).

121. Overgrote meerderheid etiketten voorzien van zwangerschapspictogram [The vast majority of labels are provided with a pregnancy icon]. The Hague: Responsible Alcohol Consumption Foundation; 2016 (in Dutch; https://stiva.nl/nieuwsberichten/overgrote-meerderheid-etiketten-voorzien-zwangerschapspictogram/, accessed 11 December 2019).

122. Código de autorregulación publicitaria [Advertising self-regulation code]. Madrid: Federacion Espanola de Bebidas Espirituosas [Spanish Federation

of Spirit Drinks]; 2016 (in Spanish; https://www.autocontrol.es/wp-content/uploads/2016/02/cčdigo-de-autorregulaciĉn-publicitaria-de-la-federaciĉn-espa§ola-de-bebidas-espirituosas-febe.pdf, accessed 11 December 2019).

123. Código de comunicación comercial del vino [Wine: commercial communication code]. Madrid: Interprofesional del Vino de España [Interprofessional Organization of Wine of Spain]; 2018 (in Spanish; https://www.autocontrol.es/wp-content/uploads/2018/12/codigo-de-comunicacion-comercial-del-vino-web.pdf, accessed 11 December 2019).

124. Código de autorregulación publicitaria de cerveceros de España [Self-regulation code for Spanish beer advertising]. Madrid: Cerveceros de España [Beers of Spain]; 2018 (in Spanish; https://www.autocontrol.es/wp-content/uploads/2016/02/c%C2%A2digo-de-autorregulaci%C2%A2n-publicitaria-de-cerveceros-de-espa%C2%A7a-cerveceros.pdf, accessed 11 December 2019).

125. Código de auto-regulação da comunicação comercial em matéria de bebidas alcoólicas [Self-regulation code of commercial communication on alcoholic beverages wines and spirit drinks]. Lisbon: Auto Regulação Publicitária [Advertising Self-regulation]; 2017 (in Portuguese; http://www.gmcs.pt/ficheiros/pt/codigo-de-autorregulacao-da-comunicacao-comercial-em-materia-de-bebidas-alcoolicas-vinhos-e-espirituosas.pdf, accessed 11 December 2019).

126. Zwangerschapslogo op drankfles komt eraan [Pregnancy logos on drinks bottles are coming]. The Hague: SpiritsNL; 2010 (in Dutch; http://www.spiritsnl.nl/nieuws/zwangerschapslogo-op-drankfles-komt-eraan.php, accessed 11 December 2019).

127. Dobrowolne znaki odpowiedzialnościowe [Voluntary responsibility signs]. Warsaw: Browary Polske [Polish Breweries]; 2012 (in Polish; https://www.browary-polskie.pl/znaki-odpowiedzialnosciowe/, accessed 11 December 2019).

128. Communicating alcohol and health-related information. In: Alcohol Marketing Regulation Report 2017. London: Portman Group; 2017:33 (https://www.portmangroup.org.uk/wp-content/uploads/2019/09/Annual-Code-Report-2017-large.pdf, accessed 6 January 2020).

129. Botterman S, De Cuyper K, Tresignie C. State of play in the use of alcoholic beverage labels to inform consumers about health aspects. Brussels: European Commission; 2014 (http://ec.europa.eu/health//sites/health/files/alcohol/docs/alcohol_beverage_labels_full_report_en.pdf, accessed 11 December 2019).

130. Bryden A, Petticrew M, Mays N, Eastmure E, Knai C. Voluntary agreements between government and business: a scoping review of the literature with specific reference to the Public Health Responsibility Deal. Health Policy. 2013;110(2–3):186–97. doi: 10.1016/j.healthpol.2013.02.009.

131. Heineken Holding NV annual report 2018. Amsterdam: Heineken Holding NV; 2018 (https://www.theheinekencompany.com/-/media/Websites/TheHEINEKENCompany/Downloads/PDF/Annual-Report-2018/Heineken-Holding-NV-2018-Annual-Report.ashx, accessed 11 December 2019).

132. Carlsberg sustainability report 2018. Copenhagen: Carlsberg A/S; 2019 (https://carlsberggroup.com/media/28929/carlsberg-sustainability-report-2018.pdf, accessed 11 December 2019).

133. Beer wisdom [website]. Brussels: The Brewers of Europe; 2019 (https://beerwisdom.eu/, accessed 11 December 2019).

134. Anheuser-Busch InBev. Commitments to the European Alcohol and Health Forum: results 2012–2014. 2014.

135. Presence of responsible drinking messages in packaging and advertising: compliance monitoring report. Woking: SAB Miller; 2014 (https://www.ab-inbev.com/content/dam/universaltemplate/ab-inbev/investors/sabmiller/reports/other-reports/labelling-informing-marketing-commitment-report-2014.pdf, 6 January 2020).

136. Consultation on options for improving information on the labels of alcoholic drinks to support consumers to make healthier choices in the UK. London: Department of Health; 2010 (https://webarchive.nationalarchives.gov.uk/20110321200423/http://www.dh.gov.uk/prod_consum_dh/groups/dh_digitalassets/documents/digitalasset/dh_125097.pdf, accessed 11 December 2019).

137. Safe. Sensible. Social. The next steps in the National Alcohol Strategy. London: HM Government; 2007 (https://webarchive.nationalarchives.gov.uk/20130124035930/http://www.dh.gov.uk/prod_consum_dh/groups/dh_digitalassets/@dh/@en/documents/digitalasset/dh_075219.pdf, accessed 11 December 2019).

138. Tackling harmful alcohol use: economics and public health policy. Paris: OECD Publishing; 2015 (http://www.oecd-ilibrary.org/social-issues-migration-health/tackling-harmful-alcohol-use_9789264181069-en, accessed 11 December 2019).

139. Monitoring implementation of Alcohol Labelling Regime (including advice to women on alcohol and pregnancy). Chipping Campden: Campden &

Chorleywood Food Research Association Group; 2008 (https://webarchive.nationalarchives.gov.uk/20120106040909/http://www.dh.gov.uk/prod_consum_dh/groups/dh_digitalassets/documents/digitalasset/dh_091381.pdf, accessed 11 December 2019).

140. Monitoring implementation of Alcohol Labelling Regime Stage 2 (including advice to women on alcohol and pregnancy). Chipping Campden: Campden BRI; 2009 (https://webarchive.nationalarchives.gov.uk/20120106040850/http://www.dh.gov.uk/prod_consum_dh/groups/dh_digitalassets/documents/digitalasset/dh_112473.pdf, accessed 11 December 2019).

141. The public health responsibility deal. London: Department of Health; 2011 (http://webarchive.nationalarchives.gov.uk/20130107105354/https://www.wp.dh.gov.uk/responsibilitydeal/files/2012/03/The-Public-Health-Responsibility-Deal-March-20111.pdf, accessed 11 December 2019).

142. Labelling the point: towards better alcohol health information. London: Royal Society for Public Health; 2018 (https://www.rsph.org.uk/uploads/assets/uploaded/295e8a6f-56aa-4266-8362413b5f0a7c04.pdf, accessed 11 December 2019).

143. The Portman Group encourages industry to include 14 CMO units on labels. London: Portman Group; 31 July 2019 (press release; https://www.portmangroup.org.uk/the-portman-group-encourages-industry-to-include-14-unit-cmo-guidance-on-labels/, accessed 6 January 2020).

144. Right to know: are alcohol labels giving consumers the information they need? London: Alcohol Health Alliance UK; 2017 (http://ahauk.org/right-know-alcohol-labels-giving-consumers-information-need-2017/, accessed 11 December 2019).

145. Our right to know: how alcohol labelling is failing consumers. London: Alcohol Health Alliance UK; 2018 (http://ahauk.org/our-right-to-know-2018/, accessed 11 December 2019).

146. Alcohol framework 2018: preventing harm. Edinburgh: Scottish Government; 2018 (https://www.gov.scot/publications/alcohol-framework-2018-preventing-harm-next-steps-changing-relationship-alcohol/, accessed 11 December 2019).

147. Buykx P, Li J, De Matos EG, Gavens L, Hooper L, Ward B et al. Factors associated with public support for alcohol policy in England: a population-based survey. Lancet. 2016;388(S31). doi: https://doi.org/10.1016/S0140-6736(16)32267-X.

148. Astrauskiene A. Alcohol control policy in Lithuania: historical approach. Brussels: European Commission Think Before Drink Lifelong Learning Programme; 2014 (http://www.thinkbeforedrink.eu/documentation/AlkoPolicy-Lithuania.pdf, accessed 11 December 2019).

149. Midttun NG. Commentary: life after big alcohol policy changes in Lithuania. Türi: Nordic Alcohol and Drug Policy Network; 2018 (https://nordan.org/commentary-life-after-big-alcohol-policy-changes-in-lithuania/, accessed 11 December 2019).

150. Federal Law of the Russian Federation No. 171-FZ of November 22, 1995, on the state regulation of production and trading volume of ethyl alcohol and alcoholic drinks. Moscow: Government of the Russian Federation; 1995 (https://www.wto.org/english/thewto_e/acc_e/rus_e/WTACCRUS58_LEG_400.pdf, accessed 28 January 2020).

151. Anderson P, Jané-Llopis E, Hasan OSM, Rehm J. Changing collective social norms in favour of reduced harmful use of alcohol: a review of reviews. Alcohol Alcohol. 2018;53(3):326–32. doi: 10.1093/alcalc/agx121.

152. Public Health (Alcohol) Bill. Dublin: Government of Ireland; 2015 (https://www.gov.ie/en/publication/0a1a58-public-health-alcohol-bill-2015/?referrer=/wp-content/uploads/2016/05/regulatory-impact-analysis-public-health-alcohol-bill.pdf/, accessed 11 December 2019).

153. Butler S. Ireland's public health (alcohol) bill: policy window or political sop? Contemp Drug Probl. 2015;42(2):106–17. doi: 10.1177/0091450915579873.

154. Bello P-Y. Sanitary warnings on alcoholic beverages: French experience. In: Eurocare Policy Debate, the European Parliament, 17 September 2013. Brussels: Eurocare; 2013 (https://slideplayer.com/slide/4515394/, accessed 11 December 2019).

155. Craplet M. Alcohol policy in France: between traditions and paradoxes. Brussels: Eurocare; 2015 (https://intra.tai.ee/images/eventlist/events/27-11-15-alkokonverents_4_Craplet.pdf, accessed 11 December 2019).

156. Pierrefiche O, Daoust M. Use of alcohol during pregnancy in France: another French paradox? J Preg Child Health. 2016;3:246. doi: 10.4172/2376-127X.1000246.

157. Guillemont J. Labelling on alcoholic drinks packaging: the French experience. Paris: National Institute for Prevention and Health Education; 2009 (http://ec.europa.eu/health/ph_determinants/life_style/alcohol/documents/ev_20090217_co08_en.pdf, accessed 11 December 2019).

158. Dumas A, Toutain S, Hill C, Simmat-Durand L. Warning about drinking during pregnancy: lessons from the French experience. Reprod Health. 2018;15:20. doi: 10.1186/s12978-018-0467-x.

159. Guillemont J, Leon C. Alcool et grossesse: connaissances du grand public en 2007 et évolutions en trois ans. Évolutions. 2008;15:1–6.

160. Plan national de mobilisation contre les addictions 2018. Paris: Mission interministérielle de lutte contre les drogues et les conduites addictives (MILDECA); 2018 (https://www.addictaide.fr/wp-content/uploads/2019/01/20181212_MILDECA_DP_Plan1822_V2.pdf, accessed 11 December 2019).

161. [Order of the Ministry of Health and Social Development of the Russian Federation of January 19, 2007 No. 49 on the approval of warning labels on the consumer packaging of alcoholic products about contraindications to alcoholic beverage use]. Moscow: Ministry of Justice of the Russian Federation; 2007 (in Russian; http://base.garant.ru/12151745/, accessed 11 December 2019).

162. Leahy P. EU issued warning to government over alcohol bill. The Irish Times. 17 April 2018 (https://www.irishtimes.com/news/politics/eu-issued-warning-to-government-over-alcohol-bill-1.3463775, accessed 11 December 2019).

163. Public health alcohol bill: EU notification process. Dublin: Alcohol Action Ireland; 2018 (http://alcoholireland.ie/public-health-alcohol-bill-eu-notification-process/, accessed 11 December 2019).

164. Downing J. Alcohol bill dealt further blow by wine producers. Irish Independent. 30 April 2018 (https://www.independent.ie/irish-news/alcohol-bill-dealt-further-blow-by-wine-producers-36857140.html, accessed 11 December 2019).

165. Karlsson T, editor. Alcohol in Finland in the early 2000s: consumption, harm and policy. Helsinki: National Institute for Health and Welfare; 2009 (https://pdfs.semanticscholar.org/b191/cf0e57596b0a0e807f1dc9a8291e3af07993.pdf, accessed 13 January 2020).

166. Österberg E, Lindeman M, Karlsson T. Changes in alcohol policies and public opinions in Finland 2003–2013. Drug Alcohol Rev. 2014;33(3):242–8. doi: 10.2478/nsad-2013-0048.

167. Williams R, Alexander G, Aspinall R, Batterham R, Bhala N, Bosanquet N et al. Gathering momentum for the way ahead: fifth report of the Lancet Standing Commission on Liver Disease in the UK. Lancet. 2018;392(10162):2398–412. doi: 10.1016/S0140-6736(18)32561-3.

168. Murray F. Ireland's Public Health Bill: crucial to reduce alcohol harm. Lancet. 2017;390(10109):2222–3. doi: 10.1016/S0140-6736(17)32759-9.

169. McGee H. Inside Ireland's powerful lobbying industry. The Irish Times. 2 October 2017 (https://www.irishtimes.com/news/politics/inside-irelands-powerful-lobbying-industry-1.3240201, accessed 11 December 2019).

170. Socio-economic impacts of proposed regulations under the Public Health (Alcohol) Bill: final report to the Alcohol Beverage Federation of Ireland. Dublin: DKM Economic Consultants; 2017 (https://www.drinksireland.ie/Sectors/DI/DI.nsf/vPagesDI/Publications~the-socio-economic-impact-of-the-public-health-alcohol-bill/$File/DKM+report+on+impact+of+PHAB.pdf, accessed 11 December 2019).

171. O'Halloran M. Government alcohol bill is up against strong lobbying. The Irish Times. 31 October 2016 (https://www.irishtimes.com/news/politics/government-alcohol-bill-is-up-against-strong-lobbying-1.2838970, accessed 11 December 2019).

172. Calnan S, Davoren MP, Perry IJ, O'Donovan Ó. Ireland's Public Health (Alcohol) Bill: a critical discourse analysis of industry and public health perspectives on the Bill. Contemp Drug Probl. 2018;45(2):107–26. doi: 10.1177/0091450918768284.

173. Samuel H. Bigger health warnings on wine bottles will damage "the soul of France" warn country's top chateaus. The Telegraph. 13 July 2018 (https://www.telegraph.co.uk/news/2018/07/13/bigger-health-warnings-wine-bottles-will-damage-soul-france/, accessed 11 December 2019).

174. Avery MR, Droste N, Giorgi C, Ferguson A, Martino F, Coomber K et al. Mechanisms of influence: alcohol industry submissions to the inquiry into fetal alcohol spectrum disorders. Drug Alcohol Rev. 2016;35(6):665–72. doi: 10.1111/dar.12399.

175. Alemanno A. The HOB–vín judgment: a failed attempt to standardise the visual imagery, packaging and appeal of alcohol products. Eur J Risk Regul. 2013;4(1):101–12. doi: 10.1017/S1867299X00002877.

176. Picard A. Removing warning labels from Yukon liquor is shameful. The Globe and Mail. 2 January 2018 (https://www.theglobeandmail.com/%0Aopinion/removing-warning-labels-on-yukon-liquor-is-shameful/article%0A37459759, accessed 11 December 2019).

177. O'Brien P, Gleeson D, Room R, Wilkinson C. Commentary on "Communicating messages about drinking": using the "big legal guns" to block alcohol health warning labels. Alcohol Alcohol. 2018;53(3):333–6. doi: 10.1093/alcalc/agx124.

178. The notification procedure in brief. Brussels: European Commission; 2015 (http://ec.europa.eu/growth/tools-databases/tris/en/about-the-20151535/the-notification-procedure-in-brief1/, accessed 11 December 2019).

179. Minister for Health signs 23 sections of the Public Health Alcohol Bill into effect. Dublin: Government of Ireland Department of Health; 5 November 2018 (press release; https://health.gov.ie/blog/press-release/minister-for-health-signs-23-sections-of-the-public-health-alcohol-bill-into-effect/, accessed 11 December 2019).

180. Nordic alcohol policy report. Türi: Nordic Alcohol and Drug Policy Network; 2015 (http://www.nordan.org/report/, accessed 11 December 2019).

181. Karlsson T, Österberg E, editors. Alcohol policies in EU Member States and Norway: a collection of country reports. Brussels: European Commission; 1998 (https://ec.europa.eu/health/ph_projects/1998/promotion/fp_promotion_1998_a01_27_en.pdf, accessed 11 December 2019).

182. Pertseva E. Na spirtnom mogut poyavit'sya ustrashayushchiye kartinki [Frightening warning images may soon appear on alcohol]. Izvestia. 2 August 2018 (in Russian; https://iz.ru/752411/evgeniia-pertceva/na-spirtnom-mogut-poiavitsia-ustrashaiushchie-kartinki, accessed 11 December 2019).

183. Pertseva E. Ne polezut v butylku: spirtnoe ostavjat bez "strashnyh" kartinok Minzdrav vystupil protiv deputatskogo zakonoproekta [They won't get onto the bottle: alcohol will be left without "scary" pictures]. Izvestia. 11 December 2018 (in Russian; https://iz.ru/821403/evgeniia-pertceva/ne-polezut-v-butylku-spirtnoe-ostaviat-bez-strashnykh-kartinok, accessed 11 December 2019).

184. Korobeinikov D. "Alkogol' ubivayet": FAS odobrila poyavleniye ustrashayushchikh nadpisey na butylkakh so spirtnym ["Alcohol kills": FAS approved the appearance of frightening labels on alcohol bottles]. Riafan [Federal News Agency]. 4 December 2019 (in Russian; https://riafan.ru/1128015-alkogol-ubivaet-fas-odobrila-poyavlenie-ustrashayushikh-nadpisei-na-butylkakh-so-spirtnym, accessed 11 December 2019).

185. Michalopoulos S. EU health chief not satisfied with industry's alcohol labelling proposal. Brussels: EURACTIV; 5 June 2018 (https://www.euractiv.com/section/alcohol/news/eu-health-chief-not-satisfied-with-industrys-alcohol-labelling-proposal/, accessed 6 January 2020).

186. Michalopoulos S. MEPs ask Commission to reject industry's alcohol labelling proposal. Brussels: EURACTIV; 6 August 2018 (updated 23 January 2020;

https://www.euractiv.com/section/alcohol/news/meps-ask-commission-to-reject-industrys-alcohol-labelling-proposal/, accessed 25 January 2020).

187. Alcohol makers fail to meet consumers' expectations for on-label information. Brussels: The European Consumer Organisation; 12 March 2018 (press release; https://www.beuc.eu/publications/beuc-web-2018-009_alcohol_makers_fail_to_meet_consumers_expectations.pdf, accessed 6 January 2020).

188. Hillier D. The arguments for and against alcohol warning labels. Vice. 22 May 2018 (https://www.vice.com/en_uk/article/nekzjd/the-arguments-for-and-against-alcohol-warning-labels, accessed 11 December 2019).

189. Battaglene T. An analysis of ingredient and nutritional labeling for wine. BIO Web Conf. 2014;3:03006. doi: 10.1051/bioconf/20140303006.

190. Surrett J, Sawatzki K. Alcohol legislation and taxes in Turkey. Washington (DC): USDA Foreign Agricultural Service; 2015 (https://apps.fas.usda.gov/newgainapi/api/report/downloadreportbyfilename?filename=Alcohol%20Legislation%20and%20Taxes%20in%20Turkey_Ankara_Turkey_9-7-2015.pdf, accessed 11 December 2019).

191. Global information system on alcohol and health (GISAH) [website]. Geneva: World Health Organization; 2020 (https://www.who.int/gho/alcohol/en/, accessed 7 January 2020).

192. Steering Group report on a national substance misuse strategy. Dublin: Department of Health, Government of Ireland; 2012 (https://www.drugsandalcohol.ie/16908/2/Steering_Group_Report_on_a_National_Substance_Misuse_Strategy_-_7_Feb_11.pdf, accessed 13 January 2020).

193. Cogordan C, Nguyen-Thanh V, Richard JB. Alcool et grossesse. Connaissances et perception des risques. Alcohol Addict. 2016;38(3):181–90.

194. Priority on prevention: staying healthy for life. Paris: Ministry of Social Affairs and Health; 2020 (https://solidarites-sante.gouv.fr/IMG/pdf/pnsp_version_8_pages_anglais.pdf, accessed 13 January 2020).

195. Burton R, Henn C, Lavoie D, O'Connor R, Perkins C, Sweeney K et al. A rapid evidence review of the effectiveness and cost-effectiveness of alcohol control policies: an English perspective. Lancet. 2017;389(10078):1558–80. doi: 10.1016/S0140-6736(16)32420-5.

# ANNEX 1. SEARCH STRATEGY

## Databases and websites

Searches were performed in September–November 2018 (with updated searches in May–June 2019). Peer-reviewed documents with no language or date restrictions were identified from CAB Abstracts, Embase, HealthSTAR, McMaster's Health Evidence, MEDLINE, PsycINFO and Web of Science. Grey literature was searched using Google Chrome, OpenGray and The Grey Literature Report for papers, documents or presentations published from 2000 onwards in in Bosnian, Catalan, Croatian, Dutch, English, French, German, Italian, Montenegrin, Romanian, Russian, Serbian, Slovene and Spanish from any of the 53 Member States. Specific searches for documents in Russian were made on the platforms ConsultantPlus, CyberLeninka and elibrary.RU.

Additionally, websites of selected organizations relevant to the topic were searched using the integrated search function(s) of the organizations' publication database (if available), structured Google searches and hand-searching to ensure maximization of identified publications. Where possible, representatives of Member States were contacted to check for accuracy of obtained information and asked to provide extra literature relevant for their country. Other sources that were checked include the Eurasian Economic Commission, Eurocare, Europe Central Asia Monitoring, the European Alcohol and Health Forum (commitments section), International Alliance for Responsible Drinking and ministry of health websites (for the Russian Federation, the source was the Federal Service for Alcohol Market Regulation, which has a mandate to develop and alter alcohol policies in the Russian Federation, under the Ministry of Finance). For industry commitments, the results obtained through Google searches and the European Alcohol and Health Forum website were complemented with hand-searching websites of producers or producers' associations where commitments had been identified in previous searches.

## Search terms

The peer-reviewed literature was searched using the combination of alcohol, label, Europe (and expansions/synonyms) as follows, with minor variations according to specificities of databases.

**Alcohol**: (alcohol OR alcoholic beverage OR alcoholic intoxication OR (alcohol* adj3 (drink* or consum* or intake)))

**Label**: (label OR labels OR labelling OR health awareness OR health warning OR warning labels OR product labelling OR product packaging OR food labelling)

**Europe**: (((San Marino OR Austria OR Austrian OR Belgium OR Belgian OR Belge OR Bosnia OR Britain OR British OR United Kingdom OR (United adj kingdom) OR England OR Scotland OR Scottish OR Alba OR Wales OR Welsh OR Cymru OR (Northern adj Ireland) OR Bulgaria OR Bulgarian OR Croatia OR Croatian OR Cyprus OR Cyprian OR Czech OR (Czech adj Republic) OR Denmark OR Danish OR Estonia OR Estonian OR Finland OR Finnish OR France OR French OR German OR Germany OR Greek OR Greece OR Hungary OR Hungarian OR Ireland OR Irish OR Italy OR Italian OR Latvia OR Latvian OR Lithuania OR Lithuanian OR Luxembourg OR Luxembourgian OR Malta OR Maltese OR Netherlands OR Dutch OR Holland OR Poland OR Polish OR Portugal OR Portuguese OR Romanian OR Romanian OR Slovakian OR Slovak OR Slovenia OR Slovenian OR Spain OR Spanish OR Sweden OR Swedish) OR ((Albania OR Albanian OR Andorra OR Andorran OR Armenia OR Armenian OR Azerbaijan OR Azerbaijani OR Belarus OR Belarusian OR Bosnian OR (Bosnia adj Herzegovina) OR Georgian OR Georgia OR Iceland OR Icelandic 35 OR Israel OR Israeli OR Kazakhstan OR Kazakhstani OR Kyrgyzstan OR Kyrgyz OR Kirghiz OR Macedonian OR Macedonia OR Yugoslav OR (Former adj Yugoslav adj Republic adj of adj Macedonia) OR Monaco OR Monacan OR Montenegro OR Montenegrin OR Norway OR Norwegian OR Moldova OR Moldovan OR (Republic adj of adj Moldova) OR Russia OR Russian OR (San adj Marino) OR Sammarinese OR Serbia OR Serbian OR Switzerland OR Swiss OR Tajikistan OR Tajik OR Tadzhik OR Turkey OR Turkish OR Turkmenistan OR Turkmenistani OR Ukraine OR Ukrainian OR Uzbekistan OR Uzbekistani) OR (World health organization OR World Health Organization/ OR WHO European Region OR European OR Europe/ OR European Union/ OR ((Eastern adj Europe) OR (Western adj Europe) OR (Southern adj Europe) OR Baltic OR (Central adj Asia) OR (Northern adj Asia) OR (Commonwealth adj of adj Independent adj States) OR CIS OR (Middle adj East) OR EU))))

The grey literature was searched using a simplified version of the search strategy above (ensuring that it was sufficiently restrictive to create relevant hits) with restrictions for file types (pdf OR doc OR ppt) and the first 100 hits (10 pages) inspected:

- grey literature databases: "alcohol label*"
- Google: "alcohol label*/name of the country/" terms.

Russian language documents in ConsultantPlus, CyberLeninka and elibrary.RU were identified with the following keywords: Markirovka AND (alkogol'naya produktsiya OR alkogol' OR alkogol'nyye napitki OR spirtnyye napitki) Etiketirovaniye AND (alkogol'naya produktsiya OR alkogol' OR alkogol'nyye napitki OR spirtnyye napitki) Pravila markirovki AND (alkogol'naya produktsiya OR alkogol' OR alkogol'nyye napitki OR spirtnyye napitki) Reglament AND (markirovka OR etiketirovaniye OR etiketki) AND (alkogol'naya produktsiya OR alkogol' OR alkogol'nyye napitki OR spirtnyye napitki) Tekhnicheskiy reglament AND (markirovka OR etiketirovaniye OR etiketki) AND (alkogol'naya produktsiya OR alkogol' OR alkogol'nyye napitki OR spirtnyye napitki) Trebovaniya AND (markirovka OR etiketirovaniye OR etiketki) AND (alkogol'naya produktsiya OR alkogol' OR alkogol'nyye napitki OR spirtnyye napitki) Trebovaniya markirovki AND (alkogol'naya produktsiya OR alkogol' OR alkogol'nyye napitki OR spirtnyye napitki) Peduprezhedniye AND (markirovka OR etiketirovaniye OR etiketki) (alkogol'naya produktsiya OR alkogol' OR alkogol'nyye napitki OR spirtnyye napitki) Peduprezhedniye o vrede AND (markirovka OR etiketirovaniye OR etiketki) (alkogol'naya produktsiya OR alkogol' OR alkogol'nyye napitki OR spirtnyye napitki) Etiketki s preduprezhdeniyem AND (alkogol'naya produktsiya OR alkogol' OR alkogol'nyye napitki OR spirtnyye napitki) AND (Belarus' OR Respublika Belarus') (Kazakhstan OR Respublika Kazakhstan) (Rossiya OR Rossiyskaya Federatsiya) (Tadzhikistan OR Respublika Tadzhikistan) Turkmenistan Ukraina (Uzbekistan OR Respublika Uzbekistan).

The search results were first screened based on the title and abstract and those texts identified as potentially relevant were then read in full.

## Study selection

Two reviews assessed the title and abstracts of all studies identified in the search for relevance. A further assessment by two reviewers examined the full text of each relevant publication to identify papers for final inclusion. One reviewer also assessed the websites of the ministries of health and other relevant organizations (see above) to identify further documents (focusing on 2000 to June 2019).

Inclusion criteria were:

- analysed or described the availability, implementation and/or efficacy/effectiveness of alcohol labelling actions, programmes or polices;
- no language or date restrictions for peer-reviewed papers;

- website documents from 2000 onwards in Bosnian, Catalan, Croatian, Dutch, English, French, German, Italian, Montenegrin, Romanian, Russian, Serbian, Slovene and Spanish;
- reported qualitative or quantitative data; and
- from any of the 53 WHO European Region Member States.

Exclusion criteria were:

- did not describe availability, implementation or evaluation of alcohol labelling or information on alcohol labelling policies in the WHO European Region (one or more of the Member States);
- described other labelling topics with only reference to potential lessons for alcohol labelling; and
- did not provide any information about the practice or were opinion pieces or surveys of opinions.

Of the 6988 titles and abstracts screened after removal of duplicates, full-text assessment was carried out for 20 peer-reviewed papers and 299 grey literature documents. A final set of eight peer-reviewed and 116 grey literature articles were included in the qualitative synthesis (Fig. A1.1).

Fig. A1.1 PRISMA flowchart

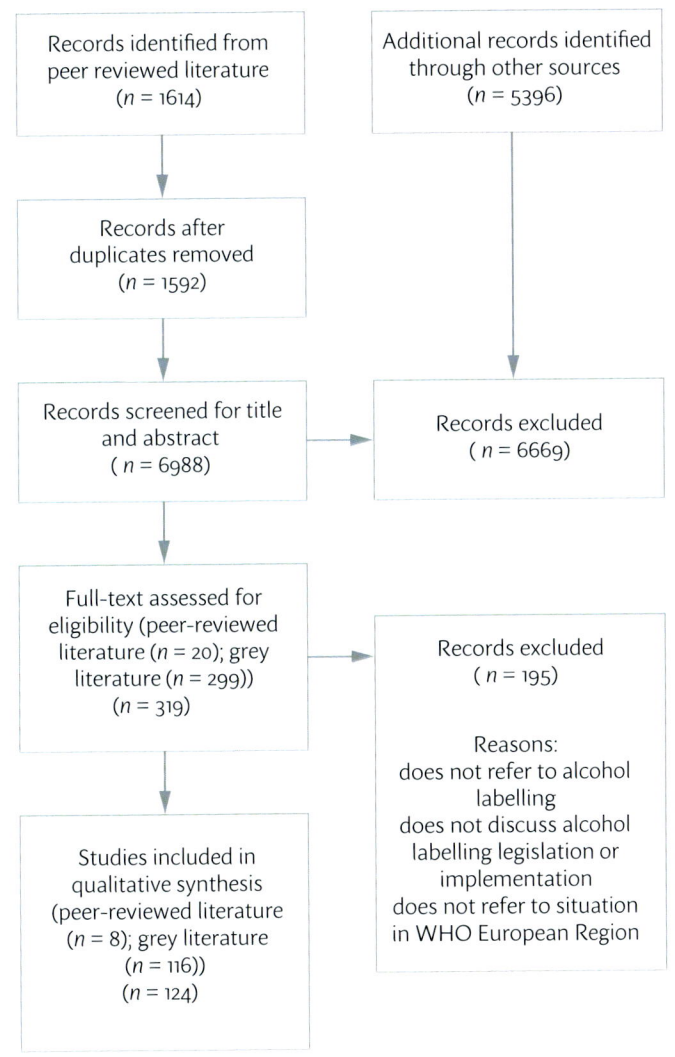

# ANNEX 2. NUTRITIONAL AND HEALTH INFORMATION LABELLING LEGISLATION AND COMMITMENTS FOR COUNTRIES AND INDUSTRIES

Tables A2.1–A2.4 summarize the information for countries and industries that was identified during the report.

Table A2.1. Nutritional information labelling legislation by country

| Country | Labelling content | Related regulations |
| --- | --- | --- |
| Armenia | IL, NV | Law of Republic of Armenia on Food Safety<br>Eurasian Customs Union Technical regulations 022/2011 on food products labelling |
| Austria | IL: sugar content for wine, ingredients for beer<br>NV: not present | Federal Ministry for Sustainability and Tourism<br>Economic Chambers, Food labelling |
| Belarus | IL, NV | Eurasian Customs Union Technical regulations 022/2011 on food products labelling |
| Bosnia and Herzegovina | IL, NV, declaration, allergens | Regulations on the provision of consumer information on foods 2013<br>Regulations on spirit beverages and alcoholic beverages 2008<br>Regulations on beer 2010 |
| Bulgaria | IL: sugar content for wine, ingredients for beer<br>NV: not present | Law on Wine and Spirits 2012<br>Ordinance on requirements for the labelling and presentation of foodstuffs 2014, 2018<br>Ordinance on the identification and marketing of wine, spirit drinks and products of grape and wine 2000 |

Table A2.1 contd

| Country | Labelling content | Related regulations |
|---|---|---|
| Croatia | IL<br>NV: not present | Beer Law Act 2011<br>Wine Law Act 2003, 2009, 2011, 2013, 2014<br>Spirit Law Act 2009 |
| Czechia | IL<br>NV: not present | Act No 110/1997 Coll., on foodstuffs and tobacco products and on amendments to certain related laws (§ 6) |
| Greece | IL<br>NV: not present | No information available |
| Ireland[a] | IL: grams of alcohol in product<br>NV: energy value in kilojoules and kilocalories | Public Health Alcohol Act |
| Israel | IL, NV | Protection of Public Health Regulations (Food) (Nutritional Labelling) 5778-2017 |
| Kazakhstan | IL, NV | Eurasian Customs Union Technical regulations 022/2011 on food products labelling<br>Law No. 429 of 16 July 1999 on state regulation of production and turnover of ethyl alcohol and alcohol products<br>Resolution No. 1081 of 20 October 2010 on requirements for the safety of alcohol products |
| Kyrgyzstan | IL, NV | Eurasian Customs Union Technical regulations 022/2011 on food products labelling<br>Technical regulations 388-2011 on beer safety, 536-2011 |

Table A2.1 contd

| Country | Labelling content | Related regulations |
|---|---|---|
| Lithuania | IL<br>NV: not present | Technical regulation for manufacturing, handling and supplying spirit drinks 2003 April 7 No. 3D-139<br>Order No. 487. Technical regulation for the description of production and production of beer |
| Norway | IL, NV[a] | Representative proposal on an offensive and solidarity alcohol policy: Document 8: 141 S (2017–2018), Settings 38 S (2018–2019) Decision 39<br>The Storting asks the Government to submit proposals to the Storting to introduce requirements for the labelling of alcoholic beverages |
| Portugal | IL<br>NV: not present | Ordinance No. 1/96 |
| Republic of Moldova | IL: for beer<br>NV: nutritional and energy information per 100 g for beer | Technical regulation of beer and drinks, based on Beer 2012, Law 1100 of 30.06.2000 on the manufacture and turnover of ethyl alcohol and alcoholic beverages |
| Romania | IL<br>NV: not present | Government decision 106/2002 (updated 2015) regarding aliments labelling (including alcoholic drinks) |
| Russian Federation | IL<br>NV: sugar content of wine | Eurasian Customs Union Technical regulations 022/2011 on food products labelling<br>Federal Law No. 171 as amended 3 July 2016, 51174-2009. Beer: general specifications |
| Tajikistan | IL<br>NV: not present | Technical regulation labelling of foodstuffs 2014 |

Table A2.1 contd

| Country | Labelling content | Related regulations |
|---|---|---|
| Turkey | IL: including additives<br>NV: not present | Turkish Food Codex food labelling and consumer information regulation 2017 |
| Turkmenistan | IL<br>NV: not present | Law on Trade 2000<br>Law of Turkmenistan on the Prevention of the Harmful Effects of Alcohol 2019 |

IL: ingredients list; NV: nutritional value.
ᵃ Legislation passed, but not yet implemented.

Table A2.2. Health information labelling legislation by country

| Country/country group | Regulation | Content of the regulation | Presentation of the message |
|---|---|---|---|
| Eurasian Economic Union (legislation common to Armenia, Belarus, Kazakhstan, Kyrgyzstan, Russian Federation)[a] | Eurasian Economic Union Technical regulation 047/2018 on the safety of alcoholic beverages, 5 December 2018 (EAEU TR 047/2018), enters into force on 9 January 2021 | A health information message "Excessive consumption of alcohol is dangerous to your health" on the container label<br><br>For consumer packaging (the box), the following health information label: "Alcohol use is not recommended for persons under the age of 18, pregnant and lactating women, as well as persons with diseases of the nervous system and internal organs" | Message should cover at least 10% of the label |
| France | Order of 2 October 2006 on implementation of Law 2005-102 Public Health Code Article L.3322-2 (Article 5 LOI No. 2005-102 11 February 2005) | Labels of beverages of above 1.2% ABV must include either the text "Consumption of alcoholic beverages during pregnancy, even in small amounts, can have serious consequences for the child's health." or a pictogram to that effect | The health information label must appear in the same visual field as the obligatory alcohol content indication, should appear on a contrasting background and should not be in any way obscured |
| Germany | Youth Protection Act | Labels of sweetened alcoholic beverages (alcopops) of between 1.2% and 10% ABV must display the following warning: "Sale is prohibited to persons under 18 under § 9 of the Youth Protection Act" | The message has to be displayed in the same typeface, size and colour as the brand or trade name or, where there is neither, as the product designation |

Table A2.2 contd

| Country/country group | Regulation | Content of the regulation | Presentation of the message |
|---|---|---|---|
| Ireland[a] | Public Health (Alcohol) Act 2018 | Labels on alcohol products will have to detail: a warning to inform the public of the danger of alcohol consumption, a warning to inform the public of the danger of alcohol consumption during pregnancy, a warning to inform the public of the direct link between alcohol and fatal cancers and details of a website, (askaboutalcohol.ie) providing public health information in relation to alcohol consumption | The Minister of Health may prescribe the form of health information labels, including size and colour, and the size, colour and font type of the printed material for each warning; and the form of the nutritional information and the website, including the size, colour and font type of the printed material |
| Israel | Regulations limiting the advertising and marketing of alcoholic beverages (Health Warning) 30 July 2013 | Labels of beverages of up to 15.5% ABV must include "Warning: Contains alcohol – it is recommended to refrain from excessive consumption"<br><br>Labels of beverages of 15.5% ABV and higher must include "Warning: Excessive consumption of alcohol is life threatening and is detrimental to health!" | – |

Table A2.2 contd

| Country/country group | Regulation | Content of the regulation | Presentation of the message |
|---|---|---|---|
| Kazakhstan[a] | Resolution No. 1081 of 20 October 2010. Technical regulations on requirements for the safety of alcohol products<br><br>In addition to EAEU TR 047/2018 | Labels of all alcoholic beverages must include the text stated in EAEU TR 047/2018 | Message should cover at least 10% of the label |
| Lithuania | Law on Alcohol Control, Art 9, Order No. 4-527 on approval of the rules for the labelling of alcoholic beverages for women in pregnancy | Labels of distilled beverages of 1.2% ABV or higher and fermented beverages of 0.5% ABV or higher are required to include a pictogram warning of the potential effects of drinking alcohol during pregnancy | Warning sign must be placed on the alcoholic container next to the other mandatory information and must be presented in a contrasting colour background so as to be clearly visible and not covered by text or other graphic symbols; diameter of the warning symbol must be at least 5 mm if the volume of the alcoholic beverage container is 500 ml or less and 10 mm if the volume exceeds 500 ml |

Table A2.2 contd

| Country/country group | Regulation | Content of the regulation | Presentation of the message |
|---|---|---|---|
| Norway[a] | Representative proposal on an offensive and solidarity alcohol policy: Document 8: 141 S (2017–2018), Settings 38 S (2018–2019) Decision 42 | Proposal confirmed by Parliament includes health information labels on containers regarding pregnancy and drinking and driving; proposal not yet in force | — |
| Republic of Moldova[a] | Law No. 124 of 12.07.2018 for amending and completing Law No. 1100/2000 on the manufacture and circulation of ethyl alcohol and alcoholic beverages | Labels of beverages of 1.5% ABV or higher must include an 18+ symbol and a symbol recommending abstinence during pregnancy | — |
| Russian Federation | Ministry of Health Decree No. 49 of 19 January 2007<br><br>Federal Law No. 218 of 18 July 2011 amending Federal Law No. 171 to include beer (previously referred only to wine and spirits)<br><br>In addition to EAEU TR 047/2018 | Labels of alcoholic beverages must contain the message "Alcohol is not for children and teenagers up to age 18, pregnant and nursing women, or for persons with diseases of the central nervous system, kidneys, liver, and other digestive organs"<br><br>Additional information as for EAEU TR 047/2018 | Message on the alcohol container should cover at least 10% of the label |

Table A2.2 contd

| Country/country group | Regulation | Content of the regulation | Presentation of the message |
|---|---|---|---|
| Turkey | Tobacco and Alcohol Regulatory Authority communiqué on warning messages to be affixed on the packaging of alcoholic beverages<br><br>Law 6487 amending miscellaneous laws and Decree Law No. 375 11/06/2013 | Labels of all alcoholic beverages must include the text "Alcohol is not your friend." and three pictograms: against drinking by minors aged below 18 years, against drinking by pregnant women, and against driving under the influence of alcohol | Warning sign must be placed on the alcoholic container next to the other mandatory information and must be presented in a contrasting colour background so as to be clearly visible and not covered by text or other graphic symbols; minimum area and dimension of the message, and the type and size of the fonts are required features that depend on the size of the product (ranging from packaging volume smaller than 100 ml, 7 cm$^2$ total area of the message and font size 6, to packaging volume greater than 1000 ml, 30 cm$^2$ and font size 12); each warning message and the total area of the warning message must be outlined in a line of flag red colour not thinner than 1 mm and not thicker than 2 mm; the message should not be obscured in any way |

Table A2.2 contd

| Country/country group | Regulation | Content of the regulation | Presentation of the message |
|---|---|---|---|
| Turkmenistan[a] | Law of Turkmenistan on the prevention of the harmful effects of alcohol (effective 1 July 2019) | Consumer packaging for alcoholic products produced in Turkmenistan (excluding products imported from other countries), including beer, low-alcohol beverages and beer-based beverages, must be marked with a contrasting warning label about the dangers of alcohol with the following content: "Alcoholic beverages are harmful to your health!", and an inscription about contraindications to its consumption as follows: "Alcoholic products are contraindicated for persons who are under the age of twenty-one, pregnant and nursing women, people with diseases of the central nervous system, kidneys, liver and other digestive organs" | Message should occupy at least 20% of the size of consumer packaging or labels; inscription should be in black upper case letters on a white background with a bold, clear, easily readable font |
| Uzbekistan | Law 302 on restriction of distribution and taking of alcohol and tobacco products 2011 Ministry of Health Regulation No. 311 of 17 November 2011 | Labels of all alcoholic beverages of greater than 1.5% ABV must include the following warning: "The excessive consumption of alcoholic beverages leads to severe diseases of the human nervous system and internal organs"; content of the warning is reviewed every five years | Message should occupy not less than 40% of the label area |

ABV: alcohol by volume.
[a] Legislation passed but not yet implemented.

Table A2.3. Industry-led commitments for nutritional information labelling

| Producer/ producer association | Pledge/commitment | Countries covered | Implementation |
|---|---|---|---|
| **Individual producers** | | | |
| Anheuser-Busch InBev | Commitment to EAHF in 2015 to share ingredients and energy information on the label for at least 80% of their volume across Europe by February 2018 and include full nutritional information (Big 7) on secondary non-returnable packaging (1) | Austria, Belgium, France, Germany, Ireland, Italy, Luxembourg, Netherlands, Russian Federation, Spain, Switzerland, Ukraine, United Kingdom | No follow-up EAHF report |
| Carlsberg | Commitment on website to place ingredients and nutritional values per 100 ml on packaging (2) | All markets | Annual Sustainability Report (2) gave the percentage of total beer volume that lists nutritional and ingredient information as 65% and 85%, respectively; specific mention of percentage of packaging with ingredients and nutritional information in western Europe (86%) on website<br><br>Methodology for deriving percentages not clear in Report or website; Report reviewed by external auditor (Price Waterhouse Coopers) with the conclusion that the data reviewed were "without material misstatements" |

Table A2.3 contd

| Producer/producer association | Pledge/commitment | Countries covered | Implementation |
|---|---|---|---|
| | | | and the Report was prepared "in accordance with the accounting policies described in the report" (2) |
| Diageo | Diageo Consumer Standards 2016 included nutritional labelling guidelines: "Including alcohol content and nutritional information per serve is minimum standard related to nutritional labelling", this applies to all single-serve containers and spirit products of 500 ml and above<br><br>Two variations of the presentation layout provided: one that uses the detailed nutritional system (per serving size in kilocalories and the Big 7 nutritional values) and one that uses the simplified nutritional system (only kilocalories per serving)<br><br>Where possible and when space allows is it suggested the detailed nutritional system should be used (3) | All markets | No information found |

Table A2.3 contd

| Producer/ producer association | Pledge/commitment | Countries covered | Implementation |
|---|---|---|---|
| Heineken | Commitment in EAHF in 2015 to provide nutritional and ingredients labelling, including energy values (kcal/100 ml) on the label for all their beer brands by the end of 2016 (4) | Austria, Belgium, Bulgaria, Croatia, Czechia, France, Greece, Hungary, Ireland, Italy, Netherlands, Poland, Portugal, Romania, Slovakia, Slovenia, Spain, United Kingdom | No follow-up EAHF report |
| | Commitment on website to provide ingredient and nutritional information per 100 ml on pack and online for all beer and cider brands produced and sold (5) | EU/outside EU | Annual Report (5) estimated that information was available for 95% of their beers and ciders worldwide in 2018 (on pack or online) Methodology for deriving percentages not clear in the Report or website; Report reviewed by external auditor (Deloitte) with conclusion that the Report was prepared "in accordance with the internally applied reporting criteria" (5) |

**Producers' associations: international**

| | | | |
|---|---|---|---|
| Group of trade associations for the European alcoholic beverages sector[a] | Self-regulatory proposal on the provision of nutritional information and ingredients listing in 2018 as a response to EC 2017 (9–13) | – | – |

Table A2.3 contd

| Producer/producer association | Pledge/commitment | Countries covered | Implementation |
|---|---|---|---|
| spiritsEUROPE | In June 2019 spiritsEUROPE signed a memorandum of understanding with the European Commission committing to providing energy values on the label and the other information (ingredients and full nutritional values) online (15) | EU-wide | No implementation yet |
| The Brewers of Europe (active beer industry body uniting 29 national associations of brewers) | The Brewers Pledge in 2012 was a commitment to the EU with a series of actions, including label information of ingredients and nutritional aspects, to be achieved by 2017 (7); in many countries, the roll-out was driven by commitments taken by the major brewers, together representing a significant share of some national markets (7) | Ingredients already listed on label: Bulgaria, Cyprus, Czechia, Denmark, Finland, Germany, Greece, Italy, Netherlands, Romania, Slovakia, Slovenia, Sweden | The 2018 Commitment Pledge (published on website) reported that "over 70% of EU beers label ingredients, with an estimated 40% also providing legally presented nutritional values (or specifically energy), predominantly on the label, complemented by digital platforms" |

Table A2.3 contd

| Producer/producer association | Pledge/commitment | Countries covered | Implementation |
|---|---|---|---|
| The Brewers of Europe (contd) | | Ingredients listing on label to be instituted in 2016–2017 with new packaging runs: Croatia, France, Ireland, Spain, United Kingdom<br><br>Nutritional values already provided: Denmark, Finland, Netherlands<br><br>Nutritional values (energy or Big 7) by 2017: Bulgaria, Croatia, Greece, Ireland, Slovenia, Sweden, United Kingdom | In 2019 the numbers were updated to 85% and 60% of the pre-packaged beers in EU labelling ingredients and calories, respectively (16); however, no further information was provided, nor on whether/how compliance was monitored; no recent industry report or independent monitoring on the implementation of this measure is available |

Table A2.3 contd

| Producer/producer association | Pledge/commitment | Countries covered | Implementation |
|---|---|---|---|
| The Brewers of Europe (contd) | The Brewers of Europe committed to including ingredients and nutritional information on their label as part of a self-regulatory proposal from the European alcoholic beverages sectors on the provision of nutritional information and ingredients listing in 2018 and announced plans to sign a memorandum of understanding with the European Commission in September 2019 to include ingredients and energy values on the labels of all beer bottles and cans in the EU by 2022 (17) | EU-wide | See above |
| **Producers' associations: national** | | | |
| Danish Brewers Association | Website states that its members have voluntarily chosen to include ingredients listing on beer, and some also include nutritional information (18); members have also committed to introduce unit labelling on their products (19) | Denmark | No information found |

83

Table A2.3 contd

| Producer/producer association | Pledge/commitment | Countries covered | Implementation |
|---|---|---|---|
| Dutch Brewers | Nutritional labelling and ingredients listing pledges at national level made in 2012 and 2015 (7,20) | Netherlands | Over a 3-year period, reported 89.3% of the beer sold on the Dutch market by Dutch brewers had nutritional declaration labels, 94.3% had information on the ingredients (7); no information on methodology available |
| Federation of the Brewing and Soft Drinks Industry | Committed in 2008 to include nutritional information on labels (8); no current information can be found on the website regarding this commitment | Finland | No information found |

Big 7: energy value plus amounts of total fat, saturated fat, carbohydrates, sugars, protein and salt; EAHF: European Alcohol and Health Forum.

[a] Comité Européen des Entreprises Vins, COPA-COGECA (Committee of Professional Agricultural Organisations and General Confederation of Agricultural Cooperatives), European Cider and Fruit Wine Association, European Confederation of Independent Wine Growers, European Federation of Origin Wines, spiritsEUROPE and The Brewers of Europe.

Table A2.4. Industry-led commitments for health information labelling

| Producer/producers' associations | Pledge/commitment | Countries covered | Monitoring |
|---|---|---|---|
| **Individual producers** | | | |
| AB InBev | Commitment to EAHF in 2011 to include pictograms regarding "no drinking during pregnancy" and "don't drink and drive" on the back labels of consumer-facing primary packaging of bottles and cans produced in Europe (2012–2014) (21,22) | Austria, Belgium, France, Germany, Ireland, Italy, Luxembourg, Netherlands, United Kingdom | Commitment report stated that 100% of bottles/cans were converted to include the pregnancy/drinking and driving pictogram in 2014 (22) |
| | Based on website information, one of the current Global Smart Drinking Goals is to place a Guidance Label on all of beer products in all its markets by the end of 2020 (23) | | |
| | Supporting public health researchers at Tufts University School of Medicine to develop a consumer guidance labelling strategy for beer to promote alcohol health literacy and reflect the current evidence base for consumer labelling (24) | | |

Table A2.4 contd

| Producer/ producers' associations | Pledge/commitment | Countries covered | Monitoring |
|---|---|---|---|
| Carlsberg | One of the responsible marketing policies states "we must make information on the potential harmful effects of alcohol available on all our alcoholic beverage packaging, using symbols, text or addresses of websites with equivalent information, in order to discourage: drinking and driving; consumption by underage persons; and consumption by pregnant women" (25) | All markets | Annual report 2018 stated that 96% of their products carry responsible drinking messages (2); no clear information on methodology for deriving data provided |
| Diageo | Diageo Consumer Standards 2016 minimum labelling requirement was to include up to three (but at least one) responsible drinking symbols related to "pregnancy, drinking and driving and underage drinking", as well as link to website with more information on "responsible drinking", applies to all packs 50 ml and above (3) | All markets | No information |

Table A2.4 contd

| Producer/ producers' associations | Pledge/commitment | Countries covered | Monitoring |
|---|---|---|---|
| Pernod Ricard | EAHF commitment to place the French pregnancy logo on the back label of all of Pernod Ricard's wine and spirit brands in EU countries by 2008 (26) | EU, Croatia, North Macedonia, Switzerland | EAHF commitment stated that all the bottles distributed in EU (as well as in Croatia, North Macedonia, Norway and Switzerland) to include the pregnancy logo (approximately 550 million bottles per year) (26) |
| SAB Miller (before the merger with AB InBev) | Two EAHF commitments: to display responsible drinking messages in all packaging and labelling of their beverages, in line with SAB Miller's voluntary guidelines (2012) (27), and to include the pregnancy responsible drinking message on at least one brand or brand variant or on a packaging type per country (2014) (28)<br><br>Responsible drinking messages to include: "Don't drink and drive", "For people over [legal drinking age] only", "Pregnant women should not drink alcohol" | Czechia, Hungary, Poland, Romania, Slovakia, Spain, United Kingdom | Monitoring found 97.5% compliance in the studied countries (Czechia, Hungary, Italy, Netherlands, Romania, Slovakia and the Canary Islands in Spain)<br><br>Reported in 2014 (28) that no examples of non-compliant labels were found, and just two anomalies identified<br><br>More detailed methodology given on how the company was reaching its EAHF commitment<br><br>Compliance monitoring for including responsible drinking messages was undertaken in 2012 with help of internal sales and marketing compliance committees in the company and reviewed by an independent external consultancy (27) |

Table A2.4 contd

| Producer/producers' associations | Pledge/commitment | Countries covered | Monitoring |
|---|---|---|---|
| **Producers' associations: international** | | | |
| Beer, Wine and Spirits Producers Commitments[a] | Series of joint commitments in 2013 to reduce the harmful use of alcohol (29), including on health information labelling: providing consumer information through the products carrying symbols or words warning against harmful drinking on their products worldwide | Worldwide | Key performance indicator was percentage of brands or percentage of volume "carrying one or more of the symbols and/or equivalent words and the address of a website containing additional information, including alcohol product strength and reminders about the dangers to health of excessive drinking" on the packaging<br><br>In the most recent report in 2017 (29): 48% achieved the indicator for companies reporting by percentage of brands; 14% achieved the indicator in companies reporting by volume (number was lower because one company could not identify the volume of its production with both symbols and a website)<br><br>Symbols or words warning against harmful drinking were present on 85% of products of the companies reporting by volume and 59% of products of companies reporting by brands |

Table A2.4 contd

| Producer/ producers' associations | Pledge/commitment | Countries covered | Monitoring |
|---|---|---|---|
| Beer, Wine and Spirits Producers Commitments (contd)[a] | | | No further methodology was given as the data depended on reports from the pledge signatory companies; despite some of the key performance indicators being reviewed by an external auditor, the labelling-related key performance indicator was not one reviewed (29) |
| **Producers' associations: national level** | | | |
| Association of Alcoholic Beverage Enterprises | Plan of declaration and self-commitment principles for consumer information and protection signed in 2005 with the leadership of the Ministry of Health and the Parliamentary Committee on Combating the Drug Abuse Problem regarding the advertising of alcoholic beverages and consumer information; member companies agreed to the inclusion of the "Enjoy responsibly" message in any advertising message communicated (30) | Greece | No information found |

89

Table A2.4 contd

| Producer/producers' associations | Pledge/commitment | Countries covered | Monitoring |
|---|---|---|---|
| Foundation for Responsible Alcohol Consumption (association of Dutch wine beer and spirit makers) | Agreement in 2013 between the industry and the Dutch Ministry of Health, Welfare and Sport that alcoholic beverage producers should be encouraged to include a pregnancy logo; voluntary introduction of the logo happened under pressure from the Government, which was influenced by the FAS-project (raising awareness of fetal alcohol syndrome) lobbying members of one of the parliamentary committees in 2011 as part of a larger EU-wide campaign; targets set for carrying the logo by 2016 – 90% of beer products, 70% of wine products and 60% of spirits (31) | The Netherlands | Internal monitoring (no information on methodology) assessed change in the average percentage of sold products with pregnancy logo from 2013 to 2016: overall increase from 21% to 89%; beer products, increase from 0.5% to 99.6%; wine products, increase from 46% to 81%; and spirits, increase from 31% to 71% (32) |
| Polish Brewers Union | Commitment in 2011 to include the combination of pictorial and written messages: "I never drive after alcohol", "18 Alcohol only for adults" and "I don't drink in pregnancy" as rotating messages on all individual and collective packaging of beer produced by breweries belonging to the Union (33) | Poland | No information found |

Table A2.4 contd

| Producer/ producers' associations | Pledge/commitment | Countries covered | Monitoring |
|---|---|---|---|
| Portman Group | Since 2011, as part of the Public Health Responsibility Deal in the United Kingdom, drinks producers representing more than 50% of the United Kingdom's market pledged to follow the guidelines issued by the Portman Group to include health information labels on their products; most recent advice is to include unit alcohol content, pregnancy logo and signposting to drinkaware. co.uk (34); further options for inclusion on the labels are low-risk weekly drinking guidelines, calorie content, drinking and driving message and logo, age-restricted product (by logo) and responsibility statement (see Case study 1) (35) | United Kingdom | See Case study 1 |
| Portuguese beer, wine and spirits producers | Code of conduct states that messages in advertising media must contain the educational reference "BE RESPONSIBLE. DRINK WITH MODERATION" (36) | Portugal | No information found |

Table A2.4 contd

| Producer/producers' associations | Pledge/commitment | Countries covered | Monitoring |
|---|---|---|---|
| Spanish beer, wine and spirits producers | A code of conduct (Autocontrol) for advertising alcoholic beverages was formulated by each sector; the beer industry pledged to put a 18+ label on all packaging in 2009; most recent editions from the wine (2018) and spirit (2013) did not include any health information labelling-related commitments, only pledging to include a moderation message on advertisements (37–39) | Spain | No information found |
| Swedish Brewer's Association | Commitment in 2007 to display one of the following messages on alcohol containers: "Under 18? Avoid alcohol", "Pregnant? Avoid alcohol", "Driving? Avoid alcohol" and "At work? Avoid alcohol" (14); no current information can be found on the website regarding this commitment | Sweden | No information found |

AB InBev: Anheuser-Busch InBev; EAHF: European Alcohol and Health Forum.
[a] AB InBev, Asahi, Bacardi, Beam Suntory, Brown-Forman, Carlsberg, Diageo, Heineken, Kirin, Molson Coors, Pernod Ricard.

# References

1. Anheuser-Busch InBev. Informing consumers about beer ingredients and nutritional values. Brussels: European Alcohol and Health Forum; 2015 (https://webgate.ec.europa.eu/sanco/heidi/eahf/commitment/view/1720, accessed 11 December 2019).

2. Carlsberg sustainability report 2018. Copenhagen: Carlsberg A/S; 2019 (https://carlsberggroup.com/media/28929/carlsberg-sustainability-report-2018.pdf, accessed 11 December 2019).

3. Diageo consumer information standards. London: Diageo; 2016 (https://www.diageo.com/en/investors/financial-results-and-presentations/diageo-consumer-information-standards-summary/, accessed 11 December 2019).

4. Heineken. Provision of nutritional and ingredients information to consumers on label for all Heineken beers in Europe. Brussels: Commitment to European Alcohol and Health Forum; 2015 (https://webgate.ec.europa.eu/sanco/heidi/eahf/commitment/view/1722, accessed 11 December 2019).

5. Heineken Holding NV annual report 2018. Amsterdam: Heineken Holding NV; 2018 (https://www.theheinekencompany.com/-/media/Websites/TheHEINEKENCompany/Downloads/PDF/Annual-Report-2018/Heineken-Holding-NV-2018-Annual-Report.ashx, accessed 11 December 2019).

6. Guinness becomes first global beverage brand to provide consumers with on-label alcohol and nutritional content. London: Diageo; 2017 (https://www.diageo.com/PR1346/aws/media/3807/guinness-labelling-press-release.pdf, accessed 11 December 2019).

7. Third report: 2012–2015. European beer pledge: a package of responsibility initiatives from Europe's brewers. Brussels: The Brewers of Europe; 2017 (https://brewersofeurope.org/uploads/mycms-files/documents/publications/2017/beer_pledge_web.pdf, accessed 11 December 2019).

8. Beer calories to be printed on labels. Helsinki: The Federation of the Brewing and Soft Drinks Industry; 2008 (http://www.panimoliitto.fi/en/beer-calories-to-be-printed-on-labels/, accessed 11 December 2019).

9. European Cider and Fruit Wine Association. Voluntary ingredient listing and nutrition information: production process for cider and fruit wine. Brussels: European Commission; 2018 (https://ec.europa.eu/food/sites/food/files/safety/docs/fs_labelling-nutrition_legis_alcohol-self-regulatory-proposal_cider_en.pdf, accessed 11 December 2019).

10. What's in a beer? European brewers' commitment to listing ingredients and nutrition information. Brussels: The Brewers of Europe; 2015 (https://beerwisdom.eu/wp-content/uploads/2018/03/whats-in-beer-20180312-1.pdf, accessed 11 December 2019).

11. Detailed wine and aromatised wine products annex to the self-regulatory proposal from the European alcoholic beverages sectors on the provision of nutrition information and ingredients. Brussels: European Commission; 2018 (https://ec.europa.eu/food/sites/food/files/safety/docs/fs_labelling-nutrition_legis_alcohol-self-regulatory-proposal_annex-wine-en.pdf, accessed 11 December 2019).

12. Self-regulatory proposal from the European alcoholic beverages sectors on the provision of nutrition information and ingredients listing. Brussels: European Commission; 2017 (https://ec.europa.eu/food/sites/food/files/safety/docs/fs_labelling-nutrition_legis_alcohol-self-regulatory-proposal_en.pdf, accessed 11 December 2019).

13. Spirits sector annex to the self-regulatory proposal from the European alcoholic beverages sectors on the provision of nutrition information and ingredients listing. Brussels: spiritsEUROPE; 2018 (https://ec.europa.eu/food/sites/food/files/safety/docs/fs_labelling-nutrition_legis_alcohol-self-regulatory-proposal_annex-spirits-en.pdf, accessed 6 January 2020).

14. Sweden to introduce booze warning labels. Stockholm: The Local; 9 July 2007 (http://www.thelocal.se/7833/20070709/, accessed 11 December 2019).

15. Consumer information: European producers sign memorandum of understanding to provide energy value on spirit drinks. Brussels: spiritsEUROPE; 4 June 2019 (https://spirits.eu/media/press-releases/consumer-information-european-producers-sign-memorandum-of-understanding-to-provide-energy-value-on-spirit-drinks, accessed 11 December 2019).

16. Proud to be clear: European brewers ahead of schedule with better ingredients and calorie labelling. In: News. 28 May 2019. Beer wisdom [website]. Brussels: The Brewers of Europe; 2019 (https://beerwisdom.eu/news/european-brewers-ahead-of-schedule-with-better-ingredients-and-calorie-labelling/, 3 March 2020).

17. All beers should be labelling ingredients and calories by end 2022. Brussels: The Brewers of Europe; 13 June 2019 (https://brewersofeurope.org/site/media-centre/post.php?doc_id=975, accessed 11 December 2019).

18. Mærkning på øl [Labelling on beer]. Copenhagen: Danish Brewers' Association; 2012 (in Danish; https://www.bryggeriforeningen.dk/ol/fodevarer/maerkning/, accessed 11 December 2019).

19. Genstandsmærkning [Object labelling]. Copenhagen: Danish Brewers' Association; 2012 (in Danish; https://www.bryggeriforeningen.dk/ol/sundhed/genstandsmaerkning/, accessed 11 December 2019).

20. Etiketteringshandleiding bij Verordening 1169/2011 [Labelling manual regulation 1169/2011]. Schenkkade: Nederlandse Brouwers; 2018 (in Dutch; https://www.nederlandsebrouwers.nl/site/assets/files/1382/handleiding_nederlandse_brouwers_bij_etiketteringsverordening_1169-2011_februari_2018.pdf, accessed 11 December 2019).

21. Anheuser-Busch InBev. Pictorial labelling commitment (submission 1323905857765-1484). Brussels: European Alcohol and Health Forum; 2011 (https://webcache.googleusercontent.com/search?q=cache:Oi5OO_0w2sUJ:https://webgate.ec.europa.eu/sanco/heidi/eahf/commitment/view/1484+&cd=1&hl=en&ct=clnk&gl=nl, accessed 6 January 2020).

22. Anheuser-Busch InBev. Commitments to the European Alcohol and Health Forum: results 2012–2014. 2014.

23. Global smart drinking goals. Brussels: ABInBev; 2019 (https://www.ab-inbev.com/what-we-do/smart-drinking/smart-drinking-goals.html, accessed 12 February 2020).

24. Tufts global alcohol labelling guidance project. Boston (MA): Tufts School of Medicine; 2018 (https://globalguidancelabel.publichealth.tufts.edu/, accessed 11 December 2019).

25. Marketing communication policy. Copenhagen: Carlsberg Breweries; 2017 (https://carlsberggroup.com/media/17989/marketing-communication-policy.pdf, accessed 11 December 2019).

26. The placement of the French pregnancy logo on the back label of all of Pernod Ricard's wine and spirit brands in the EU-27 countries. In: Annual Report 2007/2008. Paris: Pernod Ricard SA; 2008:93 (https://www.pernod-ricard.com/en/download/file/fid/8051/, accessed 11 December 2019).

27. Presence of responsible drinking messages in packaging and advertising: compliance monitoring report. Woking: SAB Miller; 2014 (https://www.ab-inbev.com/content/dam/universaltemplate/ab-inbev/investors/sabmiller/reports/

other-reports/labelling-informing-marketing-commitment-report-2014.pdf, 6 January 2020).

28. Labelling, informing, marketing: commitment report. Woking: SAB Miller; 2014 (https://www.ab-inbev.com/content/dam/universaltemplate/ab-inbev/investors/sabmiller/reports/other-reports/labelling-informing-marketing-commitment-report-2014.pdf, accessed 11 December 2019).

29. Beer, wine and spirits producers' commitments: combating harmful drinking. 2017 progress report and five-year summary of actions. London: International Alliance for Responsible Drinking; 2018 (https://www.iard.org/getattachment/61806635-0fc1-4dbb-a816-92dd167de8d1/2017-producers-commitments-full-report.pdf, accessed 11 December 2019).

30. [About the Responsibility Alliance]. Greece: The Alcoholic Drinks Association Responsibility Alliance; 2018 (in Greek; http://responsibility-alliance.gr/#members%0A, accessed 11 December 2019).

31. Zwangerschapslogo op drankfles komt eraan [Pregnancy logos on drinks bottles are coming]. The Hague: SpiritsNL; 2010 (in Dutch; http://www.spiritsnl.nl/nieuws/zwangerschapslogo-op-drankfles-komt-eraan.php, accessed 11 December 2019).

32. Overgrote meerderheid etiketten voorzien van zwangerschapspictogram [The vast majority of labels are provided with a pregnancy icon]. The Hague: Responsible Alcohol Consumption Foundation; 2016 (in Dutch; https://stiva.nl/nieuwsberichten/overgrote-meerderheid-etiketten-voorzien-zwangerschapspictogram/, accessed 11 December 2019).

33. Dobrowolne znaki odpowiedzialnościowe [Voluntary responsibility signs]. Warsaw: Browary Polske [Polish Breweries]; 2012 (in Polish; https://www.browary-polskie.pl/znaki-odpowiedzialnosciowe/, accessed 11 December 2019).

34. Communicating alcohol and health-related information. In: Alcohol Marketing Regulation Report 2017. London: Portman Group; 2017:33 (https://www.portmangroup.org.uk/wp-content/uploads/2019/09/Annual-Code-Report-2017-large.pdf, accessed 6 January 2020).

35. Safe. Sensible. Social. The next steps in the National Alcohol Strategy. London: HM Government; 2007 (https://webarchive.nationalarchives.gov.uk/20130124035930/http://www.dh.gov.uk/prod_consum_dh/groups/dh_digitalassets/@dh/@en/documents/digitalasset/dh_075219.pdf, accessed 11 December 2019).

36. Código de auto-regulação da comunicação comercial em matéria de bebidas alcoólicas [Self-regulation code of commercial communication on alcoholic beverages wines and spirit drinks]. Lisbon: Auto Regulação Publicitária [Advertising Self-regulation]; 2017 (in Portuguese; http://www.gmcs.pt/ficheiros/pt/codigo-de-autorregulacao-da-comunicacao-comercial-em-materia-de-bebidas-alcoolicas-vinhos-e-espirituosas.pdf, accessed 11 December 2019).

37. Código de autorregulación publicitaria [Advertising self-regulation code]. Madrid: Federacion Espanola de Bebidas Espirituosas [Spanish Federation of Spirit Drinks]; 2016 (in Spanish; https://www.autocontrol.es/wp-content/uploads/2016/02/cċdigo-de-autorregulaciċn-publicitaria-de-la-federaciċn-espa§ola-de-bebidas-espirituosas-febe.pdf, accessed 11 December 2019).

38. Código de comunicación comercial del vino [Wine: commercial communication code]. Madrid: Interprofesional del Vino de España [Interprofessional Organization of Wine of Spain]; 2018 (in Spanish; https://www.autocontrol.es/wp-content/uploads/2018/12/codigo-de-comunicacion-comercial-del-vino-web.pdf, accessed 11 December 2019).

39. Código de autorregulación publicitaria de cerveceros de España [Self-regulation code for Spanish beer advertising]. Madrid: Cerveceros de España [Beers of Spain]; 2018 (in Spanish; https://www.autocontrol.es/wp-content/uploads/2016/02/c%C2%A2digo-de-autorregulaci%C2%A2n-publicitaria-de-cerveceros-de-espa%C2%A7a-cerveceros.pdf, accessed 11 December 2019).